Foreword

By Tam Baillie

Scotland's Commissioner for Children and Young People

This guidance, produced by the National Back Exchange, fills a gap by responding to the call from many professionals for an authoritative piece of guidance – or a 'best practice model' drawing together all the information on moving and handling – and highlights good practice from a range of case studies.

Although intended for practitioners, the language is accessible and the guidance is beautifully illustrated without being over simplified, and the child is placed firmly at the centre of the process.

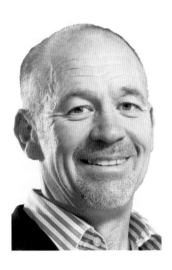

Various strategies to deal with complex handling situations are discussed and are considered from all angles, accompanied by real life case studies to allow the reader to consider all options. The point is underlined throughout that a blanket approach cannot be undertaken and that each child and each activity should be considered separately with respect for the needs of that particular child.

I am aware that moving and handling is only one of the many challenges faced by children with disabilities, but it is a very significant one. The work undertaken by my office in 2007-2008 illustrated the extent to which this dominated their lives and how important it was for them to have their views and opinions taken into account. Sadly this did not happen for many young people, the result being that they often felt anxious, disempowered and separate from the process.

Yet it was clear that most practitioners were only too aware of the need to keep the child at the centre and were keen to get this right.

They spoke of multiple barriers to implementing good moving and handling practice, not least the plethora of information available to them and what they perceived as conflicting policy and legislation. Several stated that it was not always the policy, as such, that caused difficulties but rather the variation in its implementation.

The consequence of the above sometimes led to a nervousness and uncertainty in approach which, in turn, led to an impression by some parents and carers that professionals often appeared more concerned with their own health and safety than with the best interests of the child or the wishes of parents.

I believe this guidance will assist in addressing all of these issues.

I have no doubt that such an informative source will be an enormous help to anyone working in the community with children where physical handling is required, that it will enable professionals to feel more confident in their approach and that it will ultimately lead to better practice in moving and handling which respects the dignity and worth of the child.

It comes at a time when numbers of children and young people with complex needs are rising, so the need for an authoritative source for professionals is both timely and welcome.

Although the terminology and policy context is different in Scotland and other parts of the UK, positive handling strategies – underpinned by the best interests of the child – are equally needed in all parts of the country.

I am delighted to endorse it ■

Authors' career biographies

Pat Alexander MSc, PGDip, PGCE, MCSP, CMIOSH, MIfl

Pat has worked as a physiotherapist in a variety of health care settings. These include with Dr Bobath with children with disabilities, as a back care adviser for the NHS, as well as community. She is now a free-lance manual handling practitioner and a registered member of National Back Exchange, having worked in the manual handling field since 1986.

Pat has spoken at many national and international conferences and devises courses for all levels of staff and management – and policies and risk assessments in hospital and community. She has contributed to several authoritative texts, as well as a DVD training course for Early Years staff.

Working for the HSE, among others, Pat also provides expert testimony in lifting injury cases.

Her publishing history includes:

Contributed to *Inter-professional curriculum*, (National Back Exchange 1994, 1997). 1st and 2nd edition Chapter 19 Handling Babies and Young Children in *Guide to the Handling of Patients*, 4th edition1997 (RCN/NBPA).

Risk Management in Manual Handling for Community Nurses. Contemporary Ergonomics 1998 (Taylor and Francis).

Co-author *Guidance on Manual Handling for Chartered Physiotherapists for CSP*, February 2nd edition 2002, editor 3rd edition 2008.

Co-author *Evidence Based Patient Handling: Tasks, Equipment and Interventions*. Routledge 2002.

Co-author *Standards in Manual Handling* (NBE 2010).

Co-author *Guide to the Handling of People* (5th edition) RCN/BackCare 2005, 6th Edition 2011 (in press) ∎

Carole Johnson MCSP Cert Ed

Carole is a chartered physiotherapist in the UK, working as a consultant manual handling adviser

She is a registered member of National Back Exchange, has been on the committee for a total of nine years, and is currently the public relations officer.

Her work with children spans more than 20 years; she specialises in analysis and resolution of simple and complex manual handling – showing there is often a win-win alternative.

She speaks nationally and internationally, and undertakes expert witness work.

Carole is one of the authors of *Handling of People 5th edition, 2005*, 6th Edition and of the Chartered Society of Physiotherapists' publication *Guidance on Manual Handling in Physiotherapy (2008)*.

She has also acted as an adviser and writer for a wide variety of projects and publications including:

Guidance for Safer Handling during Resuscitation in Hospitals 2001, Guidance for Physiotherapists: Paediatric Manual Handling (2010), manual handling DVD's and manual handling television programmes.

She loves both her work and 'making a positive difference' ∎

Contents

Page edge colour code where applicable

Authors: Carole Johnson and Pat Alexander

Manual Handling of Children

Caution – the publisher and authors have attempted to ensure that information in this book is up-to-date, correct and consistent with current best practice. However, manual handling practice is constantly evolving and increasing in complexity.

The information in this book is not intended to replace appropriate training and supervision. Readers should never attempt any procedure in this book without first undertaking a risk assessment. Safe handling procedures must be followed at all times. No responsibility for adverse incidents can be accepted by the publisher and authors of this book ∎

Acknowledgments

Many thanks to all those who have contributed in bringing this book to publication, their support, kindness and advice has been invaluable.

National Back Exchange

Peer Reviewers: Helen Dengel, service manager for Physical Disability Support Service for Nottinghamshire County Council for children, families and cultural services, NNEB, MSc back care management, neuromuscular approach to human movement (level 2).
Penny Townsend paediatric physiotherapist, grad dip phys, MCSP, HPC registered, manual handling adviser Kirklees Council, NBE registered member.

Publishers: National Back Exchange.

Illustrations: Elizabeth Bennett

Icon design: Jennifer Johnson

Project manager: Sue Ruszala

Project sponsor: Mike Betts

Sub-editing - design - production: Intermedia Corporate Services Ltd.

Co-operation:

Greenacres Riding school,

Stocklake Park School

Jack Tizard School,

Fairlawns Respite Centre, Kent,

Ravensbourne Special School

Liko for use of slings and hoist transfer to a horse picture ∎

Executive overview

The purpose of this book is to support anyone who works in the community with children in situations where physical handling is required.

It is hoped that it will prove useful to children and their families, as well as those who devise methods for moving and handling, employers, staff and volunteers.

Positive handling strategies are suggested and these should form the basis for facilitated discussion. It indicates where differences of opinion may lie, and suggests sources of information to help staff decide on workable solutions, from professional as well as practical viewpoints.

Various strategies are discussed for complex handling situations, with accompanying benefits and disadvantages...but each child and each activity in each setting will require an individual assessment to find the right solution for each problem. However, the task tables may inform the clinical decision making process and provide a starting point.

The legal section, and that on child-centred care, should remind all involved that movement is primarily to allow children choice and access to activities that they enjoy.

A problem solving section and blank template demonstrates the methods suggested for assessing prospective real-life tasks.

Introduction

It has been obvious for a long time that there is no authoritative source of guidance on manual handling for those working in the community with children with impaired mobility.

Advances in ante-natal and neo-natal care have improved infancy survival rates, and medical advances have improved the prognosis for many of those with life-limiting conditions – while not necessarily improving their mobility.

Hospital staff may be involved in working with very low birth weight babies and those born pre-term, who are now surviving infancy. Such children are increasing in number and are now attending both mainstream and special educational establishments.

The use of PEG feeding (Percutaneous endoscopic gastrostomy) has allowed children with swallowing difficulties to achieve their potential in size, as the nutrients are delivered by an external tube to their stomach. The increasing severity of any accompanying symptoms, such as dystonia (different tone - usually high with strong involuntary movement) has added to the need for advice and equipment to facilitate their management. Parents and handlers working in educational and respite units will need advice and training on a multiplicity of adaptations and safe work systems.

Schools and nurseries now routinely admit children with special needs, and are obliged to train a member of staff as a Special Educational Needs Co-ordinator (SENCO) or, more recently, Inclusivity co-ordinator (INCO). These people may be experienced in provision of mobility aids, but may require considerable help when assessing the needs of a highly dependent child. Added to that, many buildings are not accessible, and some may need extensive adaptations.

Many staff are struggling to ensure that children are able to access the curriculum and enjoy the same extra-curricular activities as their peers. Special seating, hoists and slings are easily available in some areas, and unknown in others. The use of the Integrated Community Stores, often with a virtual library of equipment available, does not always represent its actual state, and may result in long waits for missing parts.

Children are enjoying more adventurous activities, and inclusive education encourages them to study a greater variety of subjects. School trips and family outings demand more access for families with a mobility impaired child, and the Disability Discrimination Act 1998 (which has now been incorporated into the Equality Act 2010) has improved facilities for wheelchair users and those with sensory impairments.

However, many statutory bodies are unsure of their responsibilities, and/or require guidance in implementation. Some local authorities may have advisers who can help provide advice on accessibility to different environments.

Many wheelchairs, and some buggies, are now 'crash tested', allowing children to travel in wheelchair accessible vehicles (WAVs) safely secured in their wheelchairs. Families with children aged three and over can apply for an adapted vehicle from the Motability scheme.

This may enable a family to participate in family outings like their peers. Shopping, hobbies and holidays should not be denied to families, simply because their child is disabled. Visits to relatives should be facilitated, and may require duplication of equipment if frequent.

Many families receive no advice on manual handling, or may prefer to continue to use unsafe methods, even when equipment and guidance has been supplied. There is an anomaly that paid staff receive such training while many parents who provide care throughout the day and night, and over the years, do not.

As a result they may acquire musculo-skeletal problems which then add to their difficulties.

The timely provision of housing adaptations may enable families to continue in their present housing, or an alternative strategy of moving home may need to be considered. Advice from healthcare professionals, as well as builders, will ensure their changing needs are planned for.

This book will clearly lay out strategies to ensure these children arrive at school in a safe and timely manner, are enabled to receive the education that they require, enjoy their schooling and leisure time, and arrive home safe and happy.

It should help their families and carers, as well as therapists, support them safely and enable them to reach their planned goals.

Commonly met paediatric conditions

The intention of this section is to give a generalised overview of some of the health conditions experienced by some children. For more detailed information please refer to texts such as Hull, Johnston (1999) and Townsend (2010) as referenced on page 78.

- Genetic conditions and birth defects
- Birth trauma
- Deteriorating conditions
- Acquired trauma

Some of these conditions may be accompanied by epilepsy of varying severity.

Genetic and birth defects

Genetic-linked disorders may be due to one or both parents carrying genes which, when combined, cause a high probability of their offspring suffering from certain disorders. Other disorders may be due to genetic mutations. Some may be due to foetal exposure to environmental conditions, such as ionising radiation, various maternal diseases such as rubella or other, unknown, causes.

Downs Syndrome

Down's syndrome, causing global delay and reduced cognitive ability, may be linked to low postural tone, hyper mobile joints and heart defects. These children may require physiotherapy and occupational therapy to improve their mobility. Occasionally they may require walking assistance to achieve mobility.

Spina bifida

Spina-bifida, where there is incomplete neural tube closure in the spine and sometimes in addition an open wound on the back, may cause weakness or paralysis of the trunk or legs, depending on the level of the lesion – and may be accompanied by learning disabilities.

It may also be associated with bladder and bowel problems, and may be accompanied by hydrocephalus, requiring insertion of a shunt to prevent further swelling of the head. Should the shunts become blocked, causing drowsiness and fever, the child will require medical attention to deal with the situation.

Many of those affected are able to perform standing or slide board type transfers. Others may require hoisting. Urinary problems may require intermittent catheterisation, which will have implications of privacy, height-adjustable changing tables and relevant training. Some may wear calipers, and use a standing frame to improve their weight bearing and maintain muscle length and joint range.

It is important to encourage as much mobility as possible and to enable the child to keep within reasonable weight limits.

Sensory impairments

Sensory impairment may appear alone, or as part of another condition. Apart from communication problems, these may lead to relationship and other social disorders. These will need to be taken into account when assisting with transfers.

Autisitic spectrum disorders

Children with disorders on the autistic spectrum may have difficulty with communication and relationships. Problems will vary with the severity of the disorder, from children with Aspergers to those with more severe problems on the spectrum, or classic autism.

Physical manifestations may vary from walking problems to challenging behaviour. Children "on the spectrum" may, of course, also suffer from physical diseases – thus making any manual handling more complex.

Less common conditions

The following summary is simply an introduction to the manual handling problems which may be associated with various conditions, not as a detailed account of their symptomology or prognosis.

Achondraplasia

Achondraplasia, or 'dwarfism', may be due to inherited genes or a mutation. Children may only achieve limited height, with limbs shorter than the proportions of their trunk would indicate. Their weight-bearing may be reduced due to lower limb weakness, and their environment will require modification to allow them to reach or step up far enough. Special low toilets with a low level flush may be required. Height-adjustable tables and chairs will help enable them to interact with their peers.

Later in life some may suffer cardiac or spinal problems, both of which may reduce their mobility. Selecting slings may present problems, and individually sized/tailored slings may be required.

Arthogryposis

This condition is very obvious at birth, as the infant will have contracted limbs and immobile joints. The lower limbs may be straightened surgically, but the upper limb problems may be more difficult to solve. There may be reduced dexterity and sit-to-stand difficulties, leading to problems with daily living activities. Transfer levels may be important to facilitate independence. Children may need to be fitted with a trunk brace to prevent further postural problems.

Osteogenesis imperfecta (brittle bones)

Children with this condition may be born with already existing fractures to their brittle bones, due to the birthing process.

Trivial trauma, such as sneezing, may cause later fractures of any bone, leading to considerable disability. Some children may become wheelchair users, with contractures of various joints.

Transfer problems may arise, as parents/handlers are understandably anxious about mechanical hoisting, as they believe that human arms must be softer and less likely to cause an injury.

In fact, as the weight may only be supported on the handler's arms when lifting manually, the child may be more safely supported in a well fitted sling, which will take weight wherever the body is in contact with it.

Slings are usually left in situ in the wheelchair, to reduce any unnecessary manual handling for the child.

A manual handling practitioner (MHP) may be asked to advise on emergency evacuation measures, which will be made more difficult by the potential damage that may be caused during routine practice.

Many believe that the Personal Emergency Evacuation Plan (PEEP) should be devised and practiced without physically involving the child, using a dummy or similar. In this way, a safe routine may be made familiar to handlers and child, without putting the child at risk of unnecessary fractures.

Of course it must first be established that it is a routine practice, and not a real emergency. The latter will require communication aids for staff.

Birth trauma

Lengthy labour and delivery, or indeed any interference with the blood supply to the foetus, may cause a variety of conditions in the neonate. Premature birth may also cause cognitive, sensory and physical problems.

Asphyxia or oxygen deprivation may lead to cerebral palsy, cognitive impairment, seizures or other cerebral damage.

Cerebral Palsy

This is a condition affecting neonates, either due to abnormal brain development or trauma in utero, foetal distress, prematurity or birth trauma, and may cause variations in tone and delays in achievement of developmental milestones.

Such children may have mild weakness of one or more limbs or suffer more severe symptoms in all four limbs and trunk. It may cause problems with achieving an independent sitting position, requiring seating systems to give postural stability. Some children suffer with seizures, which are usually treated by medication, but plans must be made to administer emergency medication (if required) to prevent serious neurological damage. This may require rectal medication, which will produce handling issues. Some doctors will prescribe oral medication, but such prescription is quite patchy in the UK.

Hoisting may become necessary, and special care should be taken in selecting slings, as they may require being left in situ, due to the close-fitting supportive seating often used by these children.

Some children may require 24 hour postural support systems, including supportive cushion forms to maintain a good posture during sleep. Positioning a child into the sleep system may be difficult, due to hoisting issues.

Those suffering from strong dystonic (sustained changes in tone) spasms present complex situations when they require assistance with moving and handling. When hoisted, they may 'extend' or rotate with incredibly strong muscle tone, sometimes causing them to be at risk of

coming out of the sling. Such strong spasms may be treated by medication, botox injections or intrathecal baclofen.

Less commonly they may be treated by intermittent connection to a direct brain stimulator, which affects the part of the brain causing the problem.

Consideration must also be given to supplying an 'anti-spasm' sling, which allows them to extend by a specially designed shoulder loop to attach to the spreader bar. Rather than restraining the spasm it allows it to wear itself out, and is proving useful in some cases. These slings are made by several specialist sling companies. Many children will require an extra waist strap, inside their slings, for safety.

There will be a need for frequent physiotherapy input in many cases.

This may involve other handlers performing these programmes on a daily basis on behalf of the therapist. Special care must be taken that such handlers are competent and physically capable of performing the tasks. Often the children are prescribed a standing programme, involving a difficult transfer from sitting to standing in a prone stander. This is sometimes assisted manually by using a belt, or sliding down from a raised plinth, but more often by a hoist and standing harness.

If children with severe motor disorders are to participate in school activities such as swimming or horse riding, complex planning may be required to allow for their safe handling.

School trips will require advance planning, and usually a pre-trip visit by knowledgeable staff. Many Local Authorities will have local advisers to help, but all visits must be risk-assessed before taking place.

Deteriorating conditions

There are a variety of neurological conditions which may deteriorate at differing rates and many such diseases produce several types, or levels, of disability with varying prognoses.

A child may reach their expected milestones, and then lose their abilities at a later time. Help with mobility, such as hoisting, feeding (requiring a PEG feed, directly into the child's stomach) or even with breathing (requiring mechanical ventilation) may need to be implemented. A pragmatic approach is required to plan for the resulting reduction in mobility, as many of these conditions follow a predictable pathway. The plans will need to be made in a sensitive manner, and the child given time to accustom themselves to their changing needs. Emphasis should be placed on the positive aspects of the change, such as saving energy for the activities they enjoy.

Children prone to falling, but still being encouraged to weight-bear for therapeutic reasons, may have problems in getting up. Other children should be made aware of their own limitations to help and to avoid any manual handling (APCP 1998).

Duchenne's Muscular Dystrophy

This disorder affects the muscles of young children, mainly boys, and they tend to lose mobility throughout their childhood, with many becoming wheelchair users before adolescence.

Therapists endeavour to keep such children weight bearing as long as possible, to reduce the onset of complications. Should they start to fall while walking, staff must be aware of the local falls policy. An inflatable rescue seat may prove useful to assist the child up from the ground, while still maintaining their 'peer credibility'.

Due to scoliotic changes in the spine, there may later be need for spinal surgery to insert rods to straighten the curves. Following their post-surgery return to school, it should be recognised that they will have increased in height, and may require a larger size of sling. Their spinal movements will also be limited when inserting slings, and when leaning forward to approach a table, for example at school, work or when eating.

Handlers may feel obliged for a variety of reasons to assist, beyond safe limits, with standing transfers.

Many such young people may experience difficulty with passing urine when seated, which may be due to inaccessible clothing and an unstable posture. Adaptive clothing can be purchased online from several suppliers. To enable them to open their bowels, before they require hoisting, may require the use of an electrically operated toilet raiser seat.

Many children require hoisting later in their childhood, and due to their low tone may need structured slings to ensure their comfort and ease of positioning. The children may be extremely anxious as to their seating position, and frequently ask staff to adjust their clothing or lift them back in their chairs.

Safer methods of dealing with this repositioning must be devised. Manual handling practitioners may be asked to advise on matters of safety and emergency evacuation, balancing these needs with the importance of maintaining mobility.

Spinal Muscular Atrophy

This disease is genetically linked, and varies in its severity according to the type diagnosed. It results in weakened muscles and in some children may eventually affect those used in breathing and swallowing. Thus a PEG (Percutaneous endoscopic gastrostomy) feed may be decided upon, with some children requiring assistance with clearing their secretions.

Some may require walkers, or very specialised powered wheelchairs, and other equipment to enable them to achieve mobility. An active or passive exercise regime may be prescribed to reduce the stiffness of joints or to prevent contractures forming. Due to weakness of the supporting muscles, the trunk may show scoliotic changes, requiring moulded or matrix seating systems in the wheelchair. Spinal surgery may be required later, to correct spine shape and minimise the respiratory problems which may follow.

Suitable slings to remain in situ may be required if the child requires hoisting for transfers, and particular attention must be paid to comfort and position when seated. Children may remain small but, to ensure the safety and comfort of all, staff should resist the urge to lift them manually on a regular basis.

An individual assessment will allow the correct transfer method to be prescribed.

Friedreich's Ataxia

This condition may cause an unstable gait, and eventually an inability to weight bear. Some young people may also have associated heart conditions. Children may be offered support by their class mates when walking, pushing their wheelchair or to assist after a fall. This is generally not advisable, (APCP 1998).

A physiotherapy programme may be in place, and the issues around delegation must still be considered. Using the skill level scheme (Dreyfus 1986) may allow therapists to assess the skill required for each task to be delegated. Then, if the available staff do not have the necessary skills, their management may decide to identify the measures required to achieve the competency required. Alternatively, the therapist may decide to amend the tasks to be delegated, or not delegate them at all.

Childhood cancers

During acute stages of the illness, parents must be advised on safer methods of handling their child and warned of the need to keep themselves safe and well.

Later, they may need to be taught rehabilitation or maintenance exercises, and care must be taken to ensure they are protected from their own altruism when moving and handling their child. Any respite facilities offered to the family must be able to provide the required mobility assistance.

An end-of-life situation will put great emotional and physical strain on the whole family, which may require support from external agencies.

Acquired disorders/trauma conditions

Meningitis

The acute stage of this illness will vary with the severity of the infection. Following recovery, a child may be left with residual motor disability requiring therapeutic intervention and manual handling needs varying from mere supervision for transfers or walking, to complete dependency involving hoisting.

Conditions due to trauma

Major trauma – such as those caused by falls from height, or road accidents – might involve injuries to head, trunk and limbs.

There will probably have been considerable therapy input during the victim's time as a hospital inpatient, during the rehabilitation process, which may continue following discharge.

The child may require an exercise programme on a regular basis, the application of splints, and possibly a standing regime. Recovery or maintenance will be an important part of the daily routine for some children, competing with their learning needs at school for time and concentration. Learning support assistants will be involved with meeting both needs, and individual learning plans will need to linked with a manual handling plan.

Staff must remember that few children have to concentrate to hold their heads up while learning, but some may be expected to maintain a certain posture throughout a lesson, a process which may come naturally to their peers.

Staff will require training in manual handling to deal with any other identified physical needs, which may include hoisting.

Head or brain injury due to lack of oxygen

Following such injuries due to lack of oxygen to the brain (eg asphyxia or near-drowning) there may be motor deficit, as well as cognitive, problems.

Varying tone may reduce postural stability, requiring supportive seating. Hoisting to and from such seating systems may require slings to be left in situ, and care must be taken to ensure their shape and fabric is suitable.

Therapeutic regimes may often be prescribed, and therapists must ensure that support workers are sufficiently trained – and fit enough – to carry them out.

Seizures may develop and lead to need for regular medication, as well as emergency medication to prevent prolonged seizures that could cause further neurological damage. That may be administered rectally, or by mouth. There must be a written procedure, and training, for this process and details of how long a fit can be allowed to continue before it becomes necessary, as each child has their own 'fit pattern'.

Some children may be required to wear protective helmets at all times, others only when outdoors, and some not at all. That information would be recorded in their care plan, or local equivalent. Care must be taken to provide guidance for dealing with seizures in various settings.

If a shunt is fitted to reduce cerebral pressure, care must be taken to check for increased irritability, drowsiness or raised temperature – which may indicate a blockage requiring immediate medical intervention.

Behavioural problems can arise from neurological damage and head injuries, and staff may require guidance from an educational psychologist on dealing with them. For children exhibiting challenging behaviour, staff may need training in de-escalation, break-away and procedures for removing the child from the room. This should be obtained from a recognised organisation specialising in dealing with children.

Spinal injury

Major traumas can involve spinal injuries resulting in paraplegia or quadriplegia. Some children affected in that way may require mechanical ventilation obliging staff to clean an endotracheal tube, or provide suction to remove tracheal secretions.

PEG feeding may be required with the techniques taught to staff. Special training will need to be provided for those handlers. Sometimes a carer supplied by the family will accompany the child to school or nursery, and carry out those activities.

Orthoses (splints) are often intermittently applied to maintain joint and muscle range and length, with passive movements carried out to ensure joint mobility.

Any adaptations to the home and school environment will need therapeutic input, with particular attention paid to enabling the child to do as much as they can for themselves. Special walking splints may be used, and handlers trained in applying them in a safe way.

Cerebro-vascular accident

A 'stroke' can be due to a bleed in the brain, or a blockage in the blood vessels supplying it (with possible complications eg sickle cell disease, aneurysms). Either may cause cerebral damage, leading to changes of a temporary or more permanent nature. Once the cause has been established and treated, rehabilitation will begin. The amount of assistance required for transfers will vary from child to child.

Parents and handlers may be asked to assist in exercise regimes to encourage the brain to develop, or regain, its former movement patterns.

Conditions such as sickle cell disorder are more prevalent in certain races, especially those from tropical and sub-tropical areas. Red blood cells are misshapen, perhaps causing blockages in various blood vessels. This may result in a sickle cell crisis, cause extreme pain, and require medical intervention. Such children must be allowed to regulate their activities accordingly.

Summary

This brief summary of causes of disability in children should enable handlers to understand some of the handling needs they may encounter. Each individual child with handling needs, regardless of their diagnosis, prognosis or disability, must have an individual manual handling assessment, with prescribed methods of assisting mobility. Staff will need training in basic strategies of manual handling, as well as more complex ones.

Arrangements must be made for updating of assessments, which is not necessarily seen as part of a therapist's role unless it also involves carrying out a therapeutic programme.

Employers of handlers working with children are responsible for ensuring assessments are carried out and updated. Predictable outcomes must be planned for in advance, as well as those which are unexpected. In-house staff may require more training to enable them to carry out such assessments, and sometimes input from an MHP

may be required for complex cases or where agreement cannot be reached on the best strategy.

Handlers often express concern about dealing with falling children. That issue must be discussed with the relevant people, such as the child's (if appropriate) parents, the SENCO or INCO, therapists, health and safety department and the MHP. A relevant falls policy must be followed, and handlers taught what actions are expected of them. Falls prevention is often seen as the main strategy, and interfering with a fall may cause more damage to the child than allowing it to continue.

Where there is a history of falls, handlers must be warned what to expect and the child's safety taken into account in the care plan. This could mean using a helmet, buggy or wheelchair as appropriate when outside near to roads, using a walking harness and hoist when assisting walking, or using a height-adjustable wheeled stool when facilitating walking with such a child.

Handlers must be provided with any necessary equipment to enable them to work safely with mobility-impaired children. They must also be instructed in its safe use and basic safety checks, as well as any cleaning it may require.

Although not expected to select slings themselves, they should be able to advise others when a sling is damaged or outgrown.

Child-centred approach

Focusing on any one person, group or aspect when considering safer moving and handling carries the possibility that other areas may be under-emphasised or not given the importance they deserve.

Media reports, and some high profile cases, may have left the public with the idea that devising safer moving and handling strategies has been centred on the health and well being of the handler.

It is important to emphasise that the person being assisted has always been an equally important part of the picture.

Scotland's Commissioner for Children and Young People undertook a survey of young people and their families, looking particularly at moving and handling (SCCYP 2008).

There was a strong impression that professionals and staff are more concerned with the health and safety of handlers rather than the wishes and needs of the child and family or carers.

For example:

"...a young person who used a wheelchair told me of some of the challenges she faced in everyday life. She attended a mainstream school. When her condition caused her to slide down into one side of the chair, staff would refuse to help straighten her up because it was, they said, 'against health and safety'.

"That left her in a position which she described as not just uncomfortable, but sometimes painful. She would have to phone her dad to come to the school and put the situation right." (SCCYP 2008).

Dignity and comfort for the child is paramount for their well being. The manual handling that is undertaken should always aim to maintain that.

It was never the aim of the Manual Handling Operations Regulations 1992 (HSE 2004) to STOP manual handling, and certainly such issues

have been heavily debated as a result – and in particular A, B, X & Y versus East Sussex County Council (2003) raised this very conflict.

The Judicial Review focussed on the request of the family for handlers to manually lift, weighing it, under some circumstances, against risk of injury to staff.

Justice Munby gave a pattern for consideration:

"The assessment must be focused on the particular circumstances of the individual case. Just as context is everything, so the individual assessment is all. Thus, for example:

a) the assessment must take into account the particular disabled person's personal physical and mental characteristics, be 'user focused' and 'user led' and should be part of the wider care-planning process for that particular individual;

b) there must be an assessment of the particular disabled person's autonomy interests;

c) the assessment must be based on the particular workers involved (not workers in the abstract);

(however this is not as required by the MHOR 1992, where the questions as to the capability of the worker are hypothetical – author)

d) the assessment must be based on the pattern of lifting in the particular case.

"Once the assessment has been undertaken, the next step is to balance the risks and wishes and needs of the individual.

"When the assessment of the 'impact' on both the carer and the disabled person of the range of alternatives has been made (assuming there is a range), the employer must balance the two impact assessments one against the other."

(Paragraphs 128/129 A & B v East Sussex County Council {Neutral Citation Number: [2003] EWHC 167 (Admin)}).

The full judgment includes much other useful information for further study.

The position statement issued by National Back Exchange (2003) as a result of this judgement gave clear advice to its members:

"It is important that manual handling does not lead to pain/injury of the client/patient, family or staff. It is essential that the full picture is obtained; risks are assessed and documented as part of the

complete process. To truly be a useful assessment, it must not only include the expected information on the task, the person being assisted, the environment and the person undertaking the task, but include as far as possible a measure of the risks, the context, the views of the person requiring assistance, the effect on their dignity and the effect on their ability to be part of the community. The situation must also be analysed within the context of the relevant laws, codes of practice and current research. The process should give options and plans for difficult situations that may occur, such as hoist failure, lack of equipment or problems with access. The plans should be openly discussed with all relevant interested parties, with the aim of coming to an informed agreement. If agreement cannot be reached, then further advice must be sought. The process for such circumstances should be set out in the original handling plan. It is vitally important that any of our members involved in the manual handling assessment process, training and/or advisory roles avoid making over-simplified or generalised statements on the manual lifting or assisting of clients/patients (eg a blanket ban on manual lifting).

" It is important to empower both the client/patient, and the person performing the manual handling task, to work together in partnership, with a shared respect and desire to protect and care for the health of the other. Employers and organisations in the health and social care/education sectors should devise their policies and procedures on the basis of a commitment to mutually respectful relationships between the person(s) giving the care and the person receiving the care." (NBE, 2003).

More so, probably, than in any other field the manual handling practitioner has the opportunity to be the facilitator for discussion and the person who can help the child, family and staff work together.

As the HSE states in Handling Home Care (2001): "Care that is provided either without thought for the quality of life, independence and dignity of the client or without thought for the health of the care worker is not sustainable."

The Department for Education and Skills promotes **Every Child Matters** as a shared programme of change to improve outcomes for all children and young people. It takes forward the government's vision of radical reform for children, young people and families (DfES, 2004).

The document includes five outcomes – as identified by children themselves – for local change programmes to build services around the needs of children and young people to maximise opportunity and minimise risk.

The changes needed would be delivered by local leaders working together in strong partnership with their local communities, which are likely to be further developed by successive governments.

Every child matters - aims and outcomes

Aims	Meaning of outcomes
Be healthy	Physically, mentally, emotionally and sexually healthy Healthy lifestyles Choose not to take illegal drugs Parents, handlers and families promote healthy choices
Stay safe	Safe from: maltreatment, neglect, violence, sexual exploitation, accidental injury and death, bullying, discrimination, crime and anti-social behaviour in and out of school Have security and stability and be cared for Families/handlers providing safe homes and stability
Enjoy and achieve	Ready for, attend and enjoy school Achieve stretching national educational standards at primary and secondary schools Achieve personal and social development and enjoy recreation Families/handlers supporting learning
Make a positive contribution	Engage in decision-making, support the community and environment, engage in law-abiding and positive behaviour in and out of school Develop positive relationships and choose not to bully and discriminate Develop enterprising behaviour, self-confidence and successfully deal with significant life changes and challenges Families/handlers promote positive behaviour
Achieve economic well-being	On leaving school: engage in employment, or further education or training in readiness for employment Live in decent homes and sustainable communities Access to transport and material goods while living in non-low income households Families/handlers supported in being economically active

Good moving and handling should be comfortable and help all involved to achieve their aims. The manual handling practitioner (MHP) should offer help to facilitate achieving the agreed outcomes

● Department for Education and Skills 2004 Every Child Matters: Change for Children DfES 2004, Nottingham

Legal issues

There are some key Acts of Parliament relevant to working with and supporting children. It is not the aim of this publication to cover the legislation in detail, and information on further appropriate reading can be found in the appendix.

A brief overview

Health and Safety at Work Act 1974

Human Rights Act 1998

Manual Handling Operations Regulations 1992 (as amended)

Lifting Operations and Lifting Equipment Regulations 1998

Provision and Use of Work Equipment Regulations 1998

Management of Health and Safety at Work Regulations 1999

Children Act 2004

Carers and Disabled Children Act 2000 and Carers (Equal Opportunities) Act 2004 (combined policy guidance)

Mental Capacity Act 2005

Equality Act 2010

No one piece of legislation should be taken on its own as there will always be some interaction. Sometimes, on a practical day-to-day level, it may be difficult to balance the options. The aim should always be for all those involved with a child to come to a balanced set of options – which can be changed as circumstances alter – and aim to look after the health, well-being and safety of all concerned.

Health & safety

The Health and Safety at Work Act (1974) states that an employer is responsible for the health and safety of staff and others affected by his work, but not necessarily employed by him. This Act is an 'umbrella' for many other regulations, enacted by the UK or EU law-makers.

The law, in the shape of the Manual Handling Operations Regulations (as amended, HSE 2004) requires that all hazardous manual handling tasks are avoided where reasonably practicable.

Where they are unavoidable, such tasks must be assessed, and steps taken to reduce the risks found. It is accepted that risk cannot be eliminated, so the assessment should enable advice as to safer methods to be prescribed.

Tasks must be assessed in a formal manner. It is suggested in the guidance, that the following headings are used.

Manual Handling - the 5 aspects:

Tasks

Individual Capability

Load

Environment

Other factors, including psychosocial

The aim of completing the assessment is to provide a safe system of work. Particularly when working with children who are growing, changing and having a high level of therapy input, it can be difficult to find a single answer that will work for everyone for the duration of the child's development.

This assessment must be reviewed and updated on a regular basis, or when any changes occur in the situation.

Children always start life as very light and very dependent, with expectations that they are lifted and carried. There are many complex emotions, hopes, worries and adjustments to be made when a new baby arrives, even more so if a family become aware that their child has some additional health and potential developmental difficulties.

It may be even harder for families to come to terms with the issues surrounding a child who acquires a disability or health problem during their childhood. Professional staff must be aware that the ideas and solutions they wish to implement may be beneficial, but must be considered as part of the whole picture of care for that child, family and handlers.

A useful tool to look at the broad issue of risk is supplied by the Health and Safety Executive.

Step 1 Identify the hazards

Step 2 Decide who might be harmed and how

Step 3 Evaluate risks and decide on precautions

Step 4 Record your findings and implement them

Step 5 Review your assessment and update if necessary' (HSE 2006)

Information in the task templates will contribute to making an assessment of risks related to assisting children to move and transfer.

Manual lifting

Manual lifting as defined by the (HSE 2004) means "any transporting or supporting of a load (including the lifting, putting down, pushing, pulling, carrying or moving thereof) by hand or by bodily force."

There is no law or limit preventing manual handling per se. However, the guidance on lifting and lowering, carrying, pushing/pulling and handling while standing (HSE 2004) is included with the aim of protecting the workforce. Weights in the graphic below are a threshold; lifting and lowering weights heavier than those in the diagrams requires a full assessment to be made. In other words, these figures represent a threshold for lifting in those positions. The resulting assessment may indicate no heavier weights should be lifted, or that if everything else is ideal, then the guidance figures can be exceeded.

It is usually considered unlikely that a situation can be ideal, but it is known that more than double these figures is very likely to cause serious injury – even to a fit and well-trained person. For information on the guidelines refer to Appendix 3 in the HSE guidance (HSE 2004).

Two people lifting together do not have double the ability of one but rather two-thirds of the doubled figure, due to difficulties around co-ordination and finding a suitable handhold.

Although it may be safer to lift children when they are small, it must be remembered that those working in an Early Years setting are ageing themselves, whilst the children coming in are always young and often present complex handling problems. If it is known that children will require hoisting at a later time, it is often a good idea to let them experience this early in a play setting, in order to become familiar with the process. Of course, this does not mean that handlers will cease to carry out those therapy activities advised by physiotherapists.

> **Above these weights a full risk assessment should be made. Remember, there is serious risk of injury for those lifting more than double the guideline weights.**

General risk assessment guidelines (for average size people of reasonable fitness)

● There is no such thing as a completely 'safe' manual handling operation, but working within the following guidelines will cut risk and reduce need for a more detailed assessment.

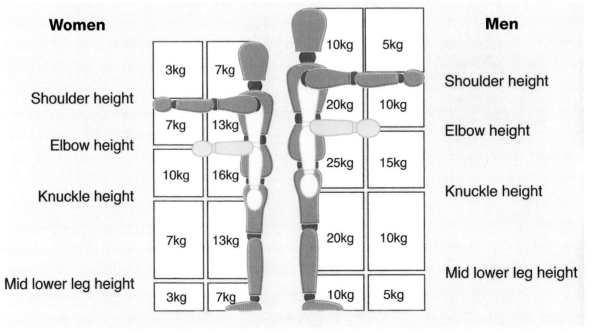

Intimate care policies

Intimate care is defined as any care which includes washing, touching or carrying out any procedure which most children would do for themselves but may not be able to accomplish because of physical disability, special educational needs, health/medical needs, or their developmental position.

In this publication the main references are for help that is given for personal hygiene. However, assistance may also be given for feeding, administration of medicines (eg rectal) and invasive procedures. Only a person suitably trained and assessed as competent should complete the task.

> Useful examples of principles when setting the policy and specific plans are listed below.

Every child has the right:

● To feel safe and secure

● To be treated as an individual

● To remain healthy

● To privacy, dignity and a professional approach from all handlers when meeting his or her needs

● To information and support which will enable them to make informed and appropriate choices

● To be accepted for who they are, without regard to age, gender, ability, race, culture or beliefs

● To information and procedures for any complaint or queries they may have regarding intimate care (Devon County Council 2006).

The policy and personal plan must be recorded and shared with the parents/guardians, and should consider encouraging independence of the child, who is the designated person to assist the child, the plan for care at school, on school trips, travelling, what to do if the designated person is not available, and where to go for advice or help when there are concerns. In addition any equipment, personal protective equipment, cleaning and disposal methods required should be documented.

Many establishments have two adults available for personal care. However care should be taken when writing policies to avoid discrimination (Equality Act 2010). An individual assessment will identify the level of support required; and if two handlers are necessary for one or more of the following reasons, it should be recorded:

■ Known record of allegation (safeguarding issue)

■ Unpredictable/challenging behaviour (as detailed in a behaviour plan)

■ They require support from two handlers for transfers (as evidenced in manual handling plan).

■ They require two handlers for medical reasons (health care plan).

This is also advisable where a child needs to be hoisted or needs physical help, but it is important to be aware that this can have an impact on the dignity and privacy of the child.

Any decision to have only one person present should be recorded and agreed with the parents/guardians and, in that situation, there should be an agreed practical process to request assistance by the person working alone.

It is important to be aware that the child is vulnerable, particularly if they are young and have difficulty communicating their wishes to the handler supporting them. Recording the child's views and wishes in a 'pen portrait' can help the handler build a general picture of the child, which can then be built upon.

The handler assisting must always be aware that the child's opinions and feelings may change as he/she grows up, and in particular when starting puberty.

The handler may have known the child for a long time, but must be sensitive to the possibility that they may no longer want a person who has known them since they were very little assisting them when they are a teenager.

It is preferable that the handler providing personal care to a young person is not teaching personal and social development to that child in lesson time.

It is helpful to consider access to facilities (eg where a child sits in a classroom and the route to the nearest facility) in order to minimise potential discomfort and time away from the activity.

Further information and links can be found at **http://www.education.gov.uk**

Practical matters - setting an evidence base

The amount of research being conducted in the physical assistance or lifting of people is only just starting to come to the fore.

In the past, the rationale for using a particular technique has been 'because an expert has deemed it the best method to use'. That choice will depend on the expert's own experience, what they themselves were taught, whether they keep up to date with research, current trends, safety bulletins, evaluation of experience and outcomes from incidents or court cases.

However, basing a suitable technique on a narrow band of information is also fraught with difficulties, and conducting research into certain techniques is full of ethical dilemmas...which leaves the handler caught in a sea of professional confusion.

The tasks in this section have been listed, as far as possible, in order of the techniques encouraging most independence.

> **Research is still limited, especially for techniques and equipment used to assist children. Expert opinion is, therefore, still the main decision-maker on which method to use.**

Certain assumptions – set out below – have been made using the tools for the tasks.

Child Size: these broad categories, developed by the authors, indicate which general size/weight of child a technique could be used for. It is important that this factor is NEVER taken in isolation.

The child size groups are:

A Babies and very small children
0-2 years, estimated weight range 3-10 kg

B Pre-school
2-4 years, estimated 11-20 kg

C Young children
4-7 years, estimated 21- 25 kg

D Older children
7-12 years, estimated 26-35 kg

E Teenagers
13-16 years, estimated 36-40 kg

F Almost Adults
16-18 years, estimated 41+ kg

Graphics: drawings illustrate possible method of undertaking a task. There are always limitations when using drawings, so please note that this can only ever be a representation.

For clarity, illustrations may not show all the details. For example, if a technique indicates that **2** are required (one handler to undertake the task and another to prepare the area, the handler preparing the area or 'blocking the view' will not be shown.

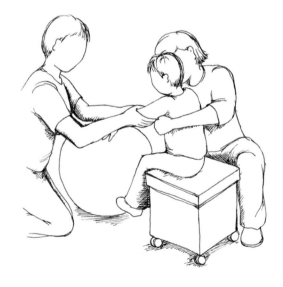

Child Ability: using the **Functional Independence Measure (FIM) (Granger et al 1993)** – this is a measure taken from a wider independence assessment tool, but has been included as it is a quick guide to the reader on the broad ability of a child in a particular situation. It must be noted that the same child may have a different FIM score for a different transfer or task. Where a score is listed, it is the range of measure of the ability required for that task.

Child ability	7	Complete Independence (timely, safely)
Child ability	6	Modified Independence (extra time, devices)
Child ability	5	Supervision (cuing, coaxing, prompting)
Child ability	4	Minimal Assistance (performs 75% or more of task)
Child ability	3	Moderate Assistance (performs 50-74% of task)
Child ability	2	Maximal Assistance (performs 25-49% of task)
Child ability	1	Total Assistance (performs less than 25% of task)

Task descriptions: these are brief descriptions to help readers understand tasks more fully. They will not contain all the possible detail for the tasks concerned.

Number of handlers: this is the minimum number of people the authors believe should be available for a task, but individual assessment and needs must determine the number of people required in each individual situation.

There may be specific situations, such as hoisting a very vulnerable child off the floor with a mobile hoist, where more handlers are needed.

The icons used in this publication are shown below:

 One handler required

 Two handlers required

 More than two handlers required

Equipment needed: this may not detail ALL the equipment required in a particular situation, but highlights the main items required and additional equipment that the reader may not have considered.

 Large equipment eg hoist or change bed

 Small, portable items eg slide sheet, handling belt

 No equipment used

Skill: this uses the Dreyfus (1986) model of acquisition of skill and has five categories, from novice to expert. If handlers do not possess these skills, their employer must ensure that they are helped to achieve them. The skill referred to is that of manual handling, and should not be used in a judgemental way.

Where two or more people are required to complete the task, it has been assumed that one person (minimum) is at the skill level indicated for that task. However, local assessment will always need to determine whether everyone needs to be at the skill level stated.

The minimum level of skill required is given for each task.

A more detailed explanation of the Dreyfus model is given, with the associated icons, below.

The Dreyfus model assumes that in acquisition and development of a skill, a student passes through five levels of proficiency: novice, advanced beginner, competent, proficient, and expert.

These different levels reflect changes in three general aspects of skilled performance. One is a movement from reliance on abstract principles to the use of past concrete experience as paradigms.

The second is a change in the learner's perception of the demand situation, in which the situation is seen less and less as a compilation of equally relevant bits, and more and more as a complete whole in which only certain parts are relevant.

The third is a passage from detached observation to involved performer. The performer no longer stands outside the situation but is now engaged in the situation. (Benner, 1984).

The 5 categories are:

Novice: a handler has no knowledge of the subject, needs clear rules and instructions to follow, and is unable to apply those rules easily to different situations. They need support and supervision.

Advanced Beginner: a handler has started to build their experience and can begin to use it in new situations.

They start to use principles, rather than fixed rules, but tend to relate everything to their own skill.

Competent: a handler has gained further insight, and can start to see the bigger picture. They may have been doing the job for a little while and demonstrate the ability to plan ahead, but do not have the speed or flexibility of the proficient handler.

Proficient: a handler shows ability to see the situation as a whole, and uses rules which are flexible in their decision making processes, which can be difficult for some less experienced handlers to fully understand. They have a good grasp of the circumstances and are efficient in dealing with the tasks required.

Expert: a handler no longer looks as if they are using rules to be able to see the whole picture. If asked how they made a decision they will tend to say that it 'felt right'. They are efficient and effective. The expert handler tends to appear intuitive.

For more detailed information please see the NBE Standards in Manual Handling (Ruszala et al 2010)

Time to complete: indicates the amount of time the authors would expect handlers to need to complete this specific task, where equipment specified for that task is in place, the right number of handlers are present, and there are no issues with behaviour or additional factors.

The time is for the manual handling part of the task only and can only ever be an estimate. Readers can estimate their times in their own situations. It can be useful to record the time taken to complete a task, as sometimes staff do not consider this aspect – which in a school setting, for example, can be of great significance. The timings have been approximated and should not be used in a competitive manner, but as a basis for discussion.

Less than
a minute

One to two
minutes

Two to Five
minutes

Five to ten
minutes

More than
ten minutes

Comfort of the child: a 10 point scale (Likert 1932 and Critchon 2001) is used to either ask the child themselves how comfortable they are when the handling task is being done or, if the child is not able to communicate that in ways the handler can understand, it may still be helpful to estimate the comfort based on individual information available. However, great care must be taken by the assessor, not to simply guess, but to use objective markers wherever possible. This may include the usual demeanour of the child at rest, facial expressions and noises during and after the task, or by comparison with other tasks for example. Please note that the aim is always to keep the child safe – as well as comfortable – while still encouraging independence.

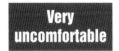 Very uncomfortable   1   2   3   4   5   6   7   8   9   10   Very comfortable

Perceived exertion and pain scales, Gunnar Borg, 1998

Handler effort (using the Borg Scale, Borg 1998): this tool was originally developed as a measurement of perceived effort and pain. It is not a linear scale – and it is possible that the longer the task takes the greater is the perception of the effort required. However, it can be a useful and simple tool for staff to measure how hard they find a task.

6	least effort	**11**	fairly light	**16**	
7	very, very light	**12**		**17**	very hard
8		**13**	somewhat hard	**18**	
9	very light	**14**		**19**	very, very hard
10		**15**	hard	**20**	maximum effort

Body Map (USDAW 2009): this uses an outline diagram of the body and coloured areas to indicate current or previous discomfort areas. In this publication it has been adapted for use for past, present or predicted areas of discomfort. It is not precise, but may help handlers allocate time to raising awareness of their own posture, or the effects of undertaking a task from a discomfort perspective.

Red is used in this publication to denote potential areas of aches and pains. If the table is being used where someone has already experienced pain, the following colour scheme can be used:

- Orange – aches and pains (not debilitating, and usually gone a few hours after the shift)

- Green – symptoms of pins and needles, numbness, shooting pains

- Blue – continuous muscle pains (ie pain which does not go away even when away from work for a day or two)

- Red – predicted areas of pain/discomfort.

Handler Risk Indicator (NPSA, 2008):

This gives an overall picture of perceived risk to the handler, using likelihood and consequences to create the matrix. For simplicity and clarity, in this book, the matrix has been used to indicate the handler's risk of injury, with the comfort scale used for the child.

But assessors are likely to find this tool very useful to look at the risk of injury to the child, especially when trying to make a balanced decision on which method to use.

Likelihood	Consequences				
	Negligible (no injury or very minor injury requiring no treatment)	Minor (minimal short term injury with minimal treatment)	Moderate (injury requiring short term treatment)	Major (injury needing longer term or significant treatment)	Severe/catastrophic (long term significant irreversible effects)
Almost certain	Low	Medium	High	Very high	Very high
Likely	Low	Medium	High	High	Very high
Possible	Low	Medium	Medium	High	High
Unlikely	Low	Low	Medium	Medium	High
Rare	Low	Low	Medium	Medium	High

Where the risk level is indicated, the perceived risk is the authors' assessment of the minimum risk. The risk may be higher in any particular situation depending on circumstances.

Considerations: in any individual situation there will be specific considerations relating to the health and abilities of the child, capabilities of handlers, the task and the environment. This section aims to flag-up areas the authors have identified which may not always be obvious to staff working in a particular situation...but it is not meant to be an exclusive list.

Alternatives: This list identifies some possible alternatives for that task. The list is not exhaustive.

> The data is there to help you. Remember you can always collect your own using the tools.

Practical moving and handling

This section looks at the practical moving and handling techniques often used with children. The techniques must only be used within the wider context of an individual manual handling risk assessment, while balancing the needs of all concerned.

Each technique table will display information relevant to that technique, including whether it is considered best practice – or whether it should be used only with caution and where specific needs arise.

There are many ways of listing techniques. The tasks in this section have been listed as far as possible from those techniques in the order of those which encourage the most independence. However, as children are often thought of in terms of their size and weight, the techniques will be detailed using this information early on in the task itself.

It is an expectation of the authors that readers will compare methods to find the best for a situation, depending on the wider information they will have for a particular child.

For example the technique of lifting a small child onto a change table with two people, one lifting the torso and one lifting the legs, is considered by many practitioners as poor practice and not a first choice method, but there may be circumstances where that method is the best interim option in that situation – and the aim is to give readers as much information as possible before needing to make a transfer.

As children grow, the handling methods appropriate to them will change. Each technique will give an indication of which general group of children this method could be used with.

Any attempt to group children will always present problems as there are children who do not easily fit into a category, and it must always be remembered that any grouping on its own cannot provide the whole picture.

Children, unlike adults, may use a number of different techniques to assist the same transfers. For some transfers they may use a hoist and for others may be manually lifted or supported. Therapy may be intense, as often the best opportunity to maximise the child's development is in the pre-school and primary school years.

As a child grows, if they need to be hoisted, the first task that is often considered for hoisting is from the floor. That requires the handler to lift through a large vertical range while supporting a child who may need extra care to hold and support. The loading on the handler's back can be significant.

> Tasks in this section have been grouped under activities, such as personal care, each category starts with those which require least assistance.

Note: The authors acknowledge that the tables in the Appendix (pages 72-77) are not exhaustive. Not all possible techniques have been included. This is a practical handbook focusing on those techniques which are most likely to be of use to practitioners.

DIY assessment template

Use photocopies of this page to complete assessments of your own tasks, using tools listed in this book.

● No responsibility accepted by the authors for data collected by readers/users.

© National Back Exchange 2011

Child's name _____

School /venue _____

Task name & brief description

Task picture
(if allowed)

Child size
(table page 20)
circle as appropriate

A B C D E F

Equipment needed
(circle and list)

Number of people
(circle)
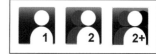

Skill required
(see page 22)

Time needed
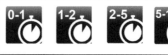

Body map (handler)
mark on outline using colour key below

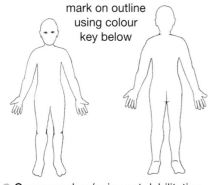

● **Orange:** aches/pains not debilitating, usually gone a few hours after shift
● **Green:** symptoms pins/needles & numbness/shooting pains
● **Blue:** continuous muscle pain which does not go away even when off work for a day or two
● **Red:** predicted areas pain/discomfort

10 = very comfortable

Child comfort
(circle one)   10 9 8 7 6 5 4 3 2 1

1 = uncomfortable

7 = Independent

Child ability
(table page 21)   7 6 5 4 3 2 1

Totally dependent = 1

Handler effort (see page 23)

6 7 8 9 10 11 12 13 14 15 16 17 18 19 20

least   somewhat hard   maximum

Risk matrix   Low   Medium   High   Very high

(circle estimated level - see table page 24)

Considerations – factors making task easier/harder

Alternatives – any considered

Assessor: _____ **Signed:** _____ **Date:** _____

Equipment

Such a wide variety of equipment is used in this field that only a small part can be included here.

It is dealt with in the following groups: hoists, slings and ancillary equipment, side-lying boards/work stations, sleep systems, small handling equipment, standing frames, walking aids, wheelchairs, inchair seating systems.

All equipment should be checked for safety and cleanliness before use, and some items, eg hoists and slings, require regular checks and maintenance by a 'competent' person from outside the organisation (to eliminate bias) see Lifting Operations and Lifting Equipment Regulations (HSE 1998) and Provision and Use of Work Equipment Regulations (HSE 1998a).

It should always be remembered that, when working with children, many staff are put at risk by having to work at a lower level than they are comfortable with.

1 Hoists

Before a hoist is installed an assessment will take place, and it is always advisable to include as many stakeholders as possible in the discussions to ensure that the most suitable hoist is supplied.

A hoist can be seen as a hindrance if selection is not carefully considered. Either a mobile hoist which can be used in any room on the same level may be supplied, or a track along the ceiling. The latter eliminates the risks of pushing a hoist and child across carpets etc and reduces clutter as it does not take up floor space.

In some organisations both types are available as, should a child require hoisting from the floor in a corridor, there may not be tracking in that area. Bathrooms designed for use by mobility-impaired children should be fitted with tracking to save space.

All hoists require regular servicing, and twice-yearly safety/weight checks (see above).

Some treatment areas are also served by tracking, allowing therapists more flexibility in their use of the area. 'Room covering' tracking – allowing movement from any point in the room to any other – also makes use of an area easier for all.

Tracking allows for the safer pick-up from the floor, as many mobile hoists do not lower sufficiently to make this easy for staff.

As an interim measure, a gantry or an arch with tracking along it, can be supplied: removing need for structural fixing to the ceiling and allowing speedy erection. Although it may be bulky in a classroom, it can be used to good effect over a nursery soft play area ■

2 Slings

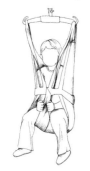

Whole body sling with waist strap

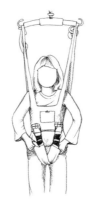

Walking Vest

Neoprene walking harness

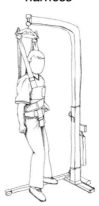

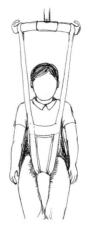

Lift pants

Slings are available in many shapes and sizes. Most children requiring hoisting have their own individual slings but occasionally, in a respite unit or an aqua-therapy pool, these may be shared. There must be clear records for each child, detailing make, size and model of sling to be used, along with any special requirements, especially which loops are to be connected to the hoist.

There has been considerable discussion about the compatibility of hoists and slings.

The easiest way of achieving compatibility is to ensure both come from the same manufacturer. If a special sling is essential for a particular child, it is advisable to check with its maker that it has been tested with the hoist it is to be used with. Confirmation from the sling supplier should be kept on file for insurance purposes.

Some suppliers will tailor a sling to fit a child with particular needs, but there are obviously manufacturing time implications involved.

Slings should always be visually checked before each use – but added to that is the LOLER requirement to have them thoroughly examined by an unbiased, competent person. This infers knowledge of hazard notices, alerts etc, as well as implications of small defects which may or may not cause problems during the next six months of use.

Children with low tone may require very supportive slings, and those with high or changeable tone may need extra waist straps and anti-spasm systems in place.

It should be noted that children with poor muscle development in the buttocks area may need particular care in sling selection, as their small dimensions may allow them to slip through some designs. The therapist, manual handling practitioner or sling-supplier should be able to advise on correct choice of sling.

The fabric may also need to be carefully chosen, due to some children requiring softer or heat-reducing material. Others may need slippery fabric to allow the sling to slide down their seat more easily or, if that is not desirable, a sling can also be temporarily inserted between two flat slide sheets already positioned under or behind the child. This makes a sling is easier to insert due to reduced friction. The slide sheets must be removed before hoisting.

Many children in moulded or matrix seating require a special sling to be left behind them in their wheelchairs. Consideration must be given to their tissue viability as to pressure problems, or friction from inserting-removing etc, together with the shape and material the sling is made of, along with ease of connecting straps to the hoist (see under Cerebral Palsy).

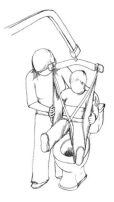

Access sling

Slings can be designed for general transfer, but can also be selected for access for toileting and dressing. However, to use a sling for toileting, users must have all four limbs, have reasonable ability to comply, sufficient muscle tone to hold their position, plus ability and motivation to keep their arms outside of the sling.

A few manufacturers supply toileting slings for children with low tone. They are secured by straps which tighten around the chest as the child's weight is supported.

A walking harness may also tighten around the chest, allowing a child to be assisted to stand by hoist. This may be included in a walking practice programme, or to access equipment such as a tricycle or stander. Other harnesses rely on straps to secure the child upright, and advice must be sought on the most comfortable and effective ones for individual children.

Repositioning in bed using hoist

A repositioning sheet can assist in turning a child, especially when used with sliding devices. Such equipment is useful if the child is in pain, is large, finds it uncomfortable to be assisted onto their side manually, has a body shape making supporting adequately by handlers difficult, or needs to be turned slowly.

Loops on one side are attached to the spreader bar and the hoist slowly raised, helping the child turn onto their side. A slide sheet may be placed under the repositioning sheet.

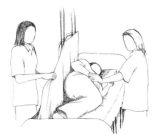

Repositioning sheet

This equipment must only be used following advice and the manufacturer's instructions. It is not suitable for all hoists. An alternative turning device has a section attached by hook and loop fastening, which can be peeled back to expose the lower part of the body for personal care – while the upper torso is still held in position ∎

3 Ancillary equipment

Turning device

An alternative turning aid which may not be suitable for all hoists or change tables, but does avoid the need for handlers to physically turn a child who has multiple-health issues. It can also enable access for personal care ■

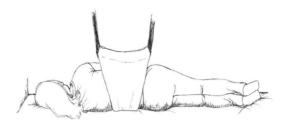

Turning device

Spreader bars

There are a number of different types of spreader bar which is the part of the hoist to which slings are attached.

The commonest types are: coathanger, four point (eg wishbone type), X-shaped, double bars, coathanger with additional side hangers, full-body suspension bars.

Each type has its own advantages for use. Before purchase of equipment it is advisable to identify the needs of the children and, when feasible, to choose options that can be interchanged where there are a wide variety of needs.

This is particularly true when using walking harnesses on standard spreader bars as they may be too wide, and mean that a small child is less comfortable or that the sling does not function correctly (Smith, 2011).

This may also be an issue for other sling types where the child uses small slings, but the spreader bars fitted are adult size ■

4 Side lying boards and work stations

These may not be very common but are useful to allow a controlled change of posture for children which need a great deal of physical support, where handlers may otherwise have a tendency to keep them in postural seating or a wheelchair.

Consideration of how the child is transferred is needed. Often the child is hoisted into the frame on their back and turned using a slide sheet, before supports and straps are secured.

If the side lying board is used on the floor, either overhead tracking is needed to hoist the child or a hoist where the legs open wide enough to reach round the equipment.

Side lying work stations are now available which can be used with a tray attached, are height-adjustable and have wheels and brakes. Those types are becoming more popular ■

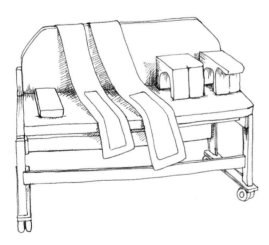

5 Sleep systems

These are available in varying types from a variety of suppliers. Basically they consist of padded supports, usually fixed to the bed or mattress to prevent damaging postures being assumed during sleep.

It can be argued that a child kept in a 'good' position throughout the day to prevent bony changes and contractures of joint structures, may then deteriorate during the night hours when unopposed muscle pull may cause joint problems such as dislocated hips.

The assessment of a child for suitability for a sleep system must be based on the health and safety of the child, as well as potential benefits. There are existing pathways detailing risks and benefits (see NW paediatric sleep system pathway and North Devon ICP etc) allowing clinicians to base their decisions on peer- reviewed systems.

Consideration must also be given to their acceptability to both child and family, including any manual handling problems arising from helping the child to bed.

When hoisting is the method of choice, a sling must be selected which allows the handler to position the child into the system, or be able to set the supports up around the child in bed.

There is sometimes a tendency for individuals to make their own adjustments – such as adding in small pillows or padding if they feel the child is uncomfortable.

It is very important that any adjustments are made by a person who has experience and a wide knowledge of sleep systems, as it is possible to introduce undue pressure on specific areas which may lead to pressure damage ■

6 Small handling and therapy equipment

Among the many aids for child-handling are those for children with ability to assist in their own transfer, as well as those for the totally dependent.

They are typically small, non-powered, items which can make the manual handling of children much easier, safer and child-friendly than it would otherwise be.

A small selection of various types are listed below in alphabetical order.

Corner seats

These are used to encourage children with tight muscles in their legs to sit with them stretched out in front and improve their sitting balance. There is often a pommel in front to encourage a good sitting position.
Corner seats often have 'outriggers' behind them for increased stability – in case the child extends backwards and tips the seat over. This reduces need for a handler to sit behind them with their own legs out in front, 'containing' the child in a 'long' sitting position which may be useful in maintaining hamstring muscle length ■

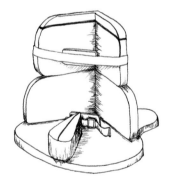

Handling belts

These broad, padded belts with handles around the waist enable handlers to ensure a safe grip when assisting a child to stand or walk.
They are not designed to lift non-weight bearing children, but are for those requiring help to rise to their feet, or those with balance problems.
Points to consider when using handling belts are: ensuring the fastening is secure, the child does not have discomfort from a stoma (artificial opening in the abdomen, often a PEG) under the belt, and that the handles are suitable for handlers to grasp. eg do not require them to stoop ■

In bed systems

These are usually take the form of a base sheet, locked into position over the mattress, with an upper sheet which can be unlocked and used to turn the child or reposition them in the bed.

They are more expensive than slide sheets – but very useful where frequent movement is required and placing a slide sheet may be uncomfortable or difficult. The number of handlers required may be reduced by using this system ■

Inflatable lifting cushions

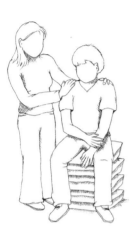

Handler and child must be trained in their use. Such cushions can be useful to assist from the floor in play or therapy, or a fallen but unhurt child.

The child can be assisted to bottom-shuffle onto the deflated cushion, or slide sheets may be used to assist them. When raised as high as required, the child can be assisted to stand ■

Kneeling 'meditation' stools

Many handlers find sitting or kneeling on the floor very uncomfortable; indeed for long periods it can increase the risk of knee damage to which handlers in Early Years settings are vulnerable.

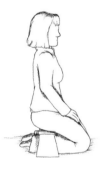

The stool is placed between the back of the thighs and calves when in a kneeling position, and reduces acute flexion at the knee as well as spreading the person's weight. If these are not available, a pillow can be used to produce a similar effect ■

Slide sheets

Slide sheets come as flat paired sheets, or as a tube, and work by reducing friction and the effort required to move a person. Some have handles or extension straps to improve grip and reduce users' need to stretch. They have a variety of uses including inserting equipment under/behind people as well as in assisting movement.

Staff should be trained in their use before attempting to move a child. Before purchase, users should consider, how the sheets will perform after frequent washing, thickness of the material, noise while using (especially if used at night) and whether the child needs a whole bed system rather than slide sheets ■

Standing frames/standers

Standers come in a variety of styles, all used to support a standing regime with all its accompanying benefits. These include reducing risk from contractures, improving circulation and respiratory movements, freeing-up the child's hands for purposeful work and possibly improving bone density – but certainly giving the child another perspective on the classroom and encouraging peer interaction.

Standers are usually prescribed by the physiotherapist, who should instruct handlers in how to assist a child into the frame.

Upright standers

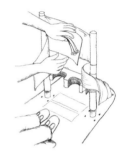

Some standers support a child, who has some trunk control, to stand upright with his/her feet at floor level. These can often by accessed by assisting a child to stand from a chair with a handling belt grasped from each side by two helpers.

Prone standers

A prone stander assists a child to remain in a slightly forward of upright position, encouraging

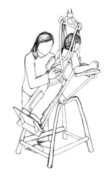

them to raise their head.

They can be used for a child with low or high tone and poor head control. Handlers often assist access to standers by a child wearing a standing harness, freeing up the handler's hands to secure the safety straps. The harness is usually left in situ when using the stander, to avoid problems of repositioning it during use.

Supine Standers

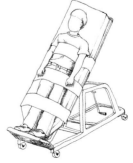

The child is usually hoisted onto these in a horizontal position, and can therefore use standard slings and hoists. Once the straps have been secured, the child is brought into an upright position. A tilt table can be used for larger children and trays can be attached if needed.

Other Standers

Less common types of standers such as self propelling standing frames may be used – for example, with children with spinal muscular atrophy and those where they start in a seated position before a hydraulic or powered system raises the child into a standing position ■

Steps

Children of diminished stature may need a step to access the toilet or the whiteboard, and to assist in many other work and play activities.

Steps can often be built up from interlocking blocks to reach the required height, or bought as fixed height units ■

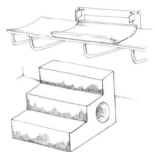

Turning discs & stand-and-turn aids

These allow a child who can weightbear – but not step around to change position – to be assisted in turning through 90 or 180 degrees.

A child requires good standing balance to use a flat turning disc. The stand-and-turn aid has a central handle rising to chest height, which the child can use to pull themselves up, and is used by the handler to turn the disc around. Children require a strong, consistent grip and arm strength to use it. Not all those available will adjust low enough for small children ■

Wedges

These may be vinyl-covered foam shapes or, sometimes, inflatable. They allow a child without sitting ability to lie face down over the high edge and put their arms down to play with toys on the floor. That can improve tone and encourage head control. Children can be positioned onto an inflatable wedge by rolling, or by hoist and harness onto the foam rubber variety.

Wheelie stools

These are often necessary when working with small children, and if adjustable enable handlers

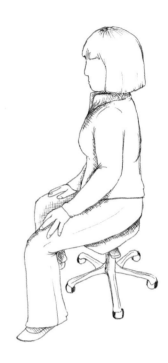

to work at a comfortable height and move around the floor by 'paddling' with their feet.

Such stools can be used to save kneeling or stooping, and are useful when assisting small children to walk.

Stable types are star-based with a small swivel top and those with a square seat and legs at the corners. Some shapes are less stable, and must be sat on astride. More recent designs have a seat back providing good lumbar support for the user.

Check the height range before purchasing, as different models vary. Users should try to avoid lifting when using these stools, and should bear in mind the Health & Safety Executive guidelines on handling loads while seated (HSE 2004).

Users should also avoid prolonged leaning down and forwards – as that may lead to strain at the base of the mobile lumbar region of the spine, where it joins with fixed bones of the sacrum ■

7 Walking aids

Walking aids include crutches, sticks and specialist items such as 'Kay' walkers. Walking frames allow a child to pull it behind them, and can have brakes to prevent it rolling back.

Using this type allows the child to approach close to a table for group work. Some walkers have a saddle provided, allowing the user to rest during their exercise.

Children can access these walkers with handlers each side helping them from sitting to standing,

and then fastening the saddle onto the frame or, depending on their abilities, by a hoist and walking harness ■

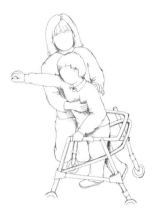

8 Wheelchairs

Some wheelchairs are designed for the user to propel by hand and some for handlers to push, while others are battery powered.

A full assessment by the Wheelchair Services is needed to determine the correct type, size and model suitable for each child or young person. Many will require a lap strap, posture belt or harness to enable them to maintain correct posture for safety and function.

Brakes must always be checked, and applied when stationary. The seat may be designed to 'tilt in space' – allowing users to adopt a more reclined position in relation to the chassis when required. Others may allow them to be raised to

their feet, and can even be used as a stander.

It is important that handlers working with a child liaise with the family and wheelchair services, so that manual handling difficulties are not inadvertently introduced at the planning stage.

A typical error might be choosing a wheelchair for a small child, who is partially weightbearing, with fixed footplates – as these often interfere with standing and result in handlers or family having to lift unnecessarily. Small children who can assist in their own transfers benefit from having a wheelchair which lowers close to floor level, allowing them independent access ■

9 In-chair seating systems

A variety of seating systems are designed for children. Clearly, if sitting balance is absent, a child will require specialised support to allow them to remain upright. That may include wings at the head, thoracic supports each side of the chest, hip supports, inclined or wedged seats, and postural harnesses. The harness may make applying a sling behind a child more difficult as, when it is released, the child's extensor thrust may bring them out of the chair. In such cases the sling is often left behind the child in their wheelchair.

Some users require a seat which

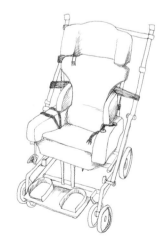

has been moulded to their shape for support. This is achieved by making a plaster mould of the user's body, or by a modular matrix system, which enables individually altered shaping should changes be required.

These seats also make it extremely difficult to insert/remove slings, hence the development by many suppliers of in-chair slings (see section on slings - page 27) ■

Simple solutions to common problems

Many problems can be eliminated if equipment supplied/provided in a special needs setting is height-adjustable. Both tables and desks, for example, can be obtained in that form.

Such adaptability reduces the possibility of furniture being incompatible, making working life much easier for handlers and children.

Equipment can take up a lot of room, whether in the home, nursery or school, and detailed planning is required when designing or adapting premises for mobility impaired people. As part of that the family, child, therapist/staff and designer should all be encouraged to give input at the relevant stages.

1 Assisting a child in the community

There are a number of places and events which children may wish to visit away from their normal environment – shopping trips, outings and respite care for example – and it would be very difficult to devise possible solutions for all of them.

From time to time manual handling may be required (see manual handling section).

The most important aspect of trips away from children's usual environments is, as far as possible, to undertake an assessment beforehand and to plan ahead...rather than having a difficult situation arise which leaves little

alternative but to perform a manual lift in much less than ideal circumstances.

Visiting the area beforehand may help, as can identifying toilet and change facilities near by that are suitable. Sometimes it is not the manual handling which is an issue, but rather pushing a person in a wheelchair over long distances (with heavy bags hanging on the chair) and rough ground, or having to use unfamiliar or different facilities.

Many issues can be solved by discussion before the trip, and a desire to find a working solution ■

2 Sitting on the floor as a treatment programme

Some treatment regimes require handlers to sit on the floor with outstretched legs behind a child, ensuring that the muscle length of the child's hamstring muscles is maintained.

Many adults find sitting in this position uncomfortable after a short time.

They should be shown alternative positions which can be used, such as leaning their backs against a wall or similar, and be reminded not to sit in any one position too long.

A kneeling stool, or cushion between the thighs

and calves, may also provide more comfort for handlers. Another strategy could be the use of a corner seat for the child.

Staff are often asked to perform stretching or assisted active exercises with children on the floor, and may find floor sitting quite uncomfortable for long periods.

Many such exercises could be assisted with the child on a height-adjustable plinth, thereby allowing handlers to stand alongside rather than having to sit on the floor ■

3 Physical Education (PE)

Staff should seek guidance from the child's therapist as to their abilities.

Educational advisors specialising in inclusivity could be asked for ideas and local facilities.

All children need to be challenged, and efforts must be made to find something they can improve at ■

4 Toileting a child unable to stand or rise unaided

There may be several solutions to toileting for a child who cannot stand or rise from a toilet seat without help.

A bottle or female urinal may be used, with a removable cutout in the seat cushion. This may also require the child to wear adapted clothing such as an extended front zip to trousers, or a drop-down front panel.

Pants with a drop-down gusset can assist a child in this activity. Alternatively, a bottle and an access sling could be used if the child has sufficient capability to use such a sling.

A rising toilet seat can help a child with weak legs. The seat may be operated by the user leaning forward, or can be electrically assisted. An assisted standing transfer could be effected with a rising wheelchair seat used in conjunction with the rising toilet seat, and would only require the handler to help with the turn.

A 'closimat' toilet – which provides a bidet type function and drying – can enable the child and facilitate a dignified approach. In that way handlers may not need to stay in an awkward posture to help with personal hygiene ■

5 Assisted walking

Some treatment paradigms require children to be on their feet when their weight-bearing ability is unpredictable.

A manual handling practitioner may advise on the

safest ways to achieve this – which may vary from the handler sitting on a wheely stool, to use of a walker or a walking harness and hoist ■

6 Swimming and aqua therapy pools

When planning a pool, competent advice must be sought from experts on the needs of the potential users. That will include the depth required, whether a slope or steps are required for access, and whether it will be at floor level or have raised sides.

Most pools for mobility impaired users require a hoist; the overhead tracking systems save room and are used often.

The changing room must be spacious, with

height-adjustable changing tables and tracking hoists, and the ambient temperature will also be important as many children with disabilities are vulnerable to cold temperatures.

Methods of evacuating a child (or staff) from a pool in an emergency must be planned, as a major seizure or choking event may occur in the water. Sufficient handlers must be dryside, as well as in the water, and a method of summoning help must be within easy reach of handlers ■

7 Handling in emergency situations

All involved in child handling will be keen to know what action needs to be taken in emergencies.

A risk assessment will inform staff of the risks involved, and the likely frequency of exposure. No one would advocate leaving a child in danger, but the organisational policies should help reduce the likelihood of such an incident occurring.

If all lessons for children with impaired mobility can be scheduled to take place on the ground floor, a Personal Emergency Evacuation Plan (PEEP) will be easier to devise.

Since the Regulatory Reform (Fire Safety) Order 2005 came into force, organisations dealing with mobility impaired people must devise a PEEP and not rely on the emergency services for assistance with evacuation.

Before that handlers were normally told to make their way to a refuge with the child, and await rescue.

Now these refuges may only be used as a temporary haven, perhaps places where a hoist can be used to transfer a wheelchair user to a stair evacuation chair.

There is no point in a handler attempting to lift a young person who is beyond their capacity, and becoming immobilised with an acute back problem at the same time.

That would simply leave two people to be rescued!

Staff must be aware of just how long the protection provided by firedoors will allow them to stay safely in certain places – and must have written plans as to how to leave the building.

If evacuation chairs are provided, there must be one for each disabled child upstairs at any one time, including library and common room facilities.

All relevant handlers and other staff must be trained in their use, and receive regular updates.

PEEPS must include emergency exit routes from all parts of the building used by children with disabilities, including when receiving personal care or using soft play areas and swimming pools.

Those children who spend time lying on a mat on the floor on a regular basis may benefit from provision of a rolled-up evacuation mat being kept close by in case of emergency.

Such mats have a stiffened, corrugated under-surface and wrap around the person, allowing them to be pulled outside more safely.

There must be plans for any foreseeable emergency in pools, such as a child collapsing, or suffering a seizure in the water.

There are several suitable stretchers which could be used, but policies must ensure that sufficient people can be summoned to deal with the situation in a timely manner ■

Finding solutions in real life

It is likely that children view moving and handling as a means to achieve an end – for example they want to go swimming, or to take part in activities with their friends.

The adults around them are likely to be thinking of a bigger picture which includes the developmental priorities of the child, safety of everyone involved, time and real-life complications, as well as the activity that the child wants to be part of right now.

Especially where a child has complex needs – or a handling task takes time, equipment and a number of handlers, and there are other children that need help or supervision – it is easy for everyone to feel that the handling is becoming an overwhelming part of the day.

If a particular procedure is followed, family or staff have predicted that in some cases there is no time to complete anything else, other than the moving and handling.

In addition it is also possible that equipment or facilities are not available or suitable for the needs of the child.

When deciding on the action to be taken where there isn't sufficient time or resources to undertake every activity according to ideal or recommended plans, strategies need to be developed which are discussed with everyone involved. Those strategies should prioritise the action, and look at alternatives while keeping a holistic perspective.

The following examples are taken from real situations to give examples of solutions. Names and details have been changed to preserve anonymity.

1 **Front standing transfer**

For a partially weight-bearing child

Environment: an adapted house with an extended bedroom, which includes an ensuite hygiene room with overhead tracking to cover the bedroom and ensuite.

The room has wide doorways, wooden floors, accessible bath, toilet with access to both sides and rails. The bedroom, living room and kitchen are all connected to a wide hallway.

The living room does not have overhead tracking or space for a mobile hoist.

The family feel strongly that they want the living room to look like a home, not an institution, and are reluctant to have equipment in that room. The settee is low and part of a suite.

Task: Sophie transfers from her wheelchair to the settee in the evenings to join her family and their dog in watching television or chatting, but has difficulty getting out of the settee when it is time to move.

Her mother tends to lift her up from the settee by standing in front of Sophie and turning her round on the spot and into the wheelchair.

Sophie is 14 years old with weakness on her left side. Finding it difficult to move her left arm and leg, she also experiences some pain in her left ankle on standing.

She is not able to perform fine motor movements with her left hand, but can reach, grip and hold on to suitably sized handles and rails.

Sophie can take up to a minute to get into a standing position, which tires her – and is easily distracted, when she tends to lose her balance.

She is very keen to enjoy weekend activities with the rest of her family, but becomes frustrated and cross when too much time is spent discussing manual handling and stopping her doing the activities she wants to take part in.

Child ability 4

Child size: **E**
Child comfort: **7**

BEFORE

Handler effort: **14**
Risk to handler: **medium**

 Child ability 5

Child size: **E**
Child comfort: **6**

AT SIX MONTH REVIEW

Handler effort: **6**
Risk to handler: **low**

Both parents feel very comfortable using this technique, although the mother noted that she has started to avoid doing this task and asking the father to help.

However, in order for Sophie's parents to have time away in the evenings, carers and volunteers may be performing the task.

One handler does not feel comfortable completing the task, one volunteer feels happy to continue with this method, but tends to twist, bend and over-reach to undertake the transfer – and another handler has been told she must not perform front transfers.

All volunteers and paid carers have received manual handling training from different organisations.

Issues: use of a technique that is likely to become more difficult as Sophie grows up.

Differing abilities and requirements for the volunteers and carers involved.

Lack of equipment that is discreet and small that the family are prepared to have in the living room.

Similar transfers have to be made in other places, particularly when Sophie is away from home.

Options investigated: following observation on how the transfer was undertaken to identify the main risks.

● Consider ways to raise the settee, which are discreet.

● Discuss with the family and physiotherapist ways to teach Sophie methods to encourage her independence.

● Consider sideways transfer into the wheelchair, after removing armrest.

● Discuss with the family trialling a turning device which can be easily moved and stored in the bedroom.

Outcome

● The turning device having been accepted in the short term.

● Sophie practiced sit-to-stand, encouraging patterns of movement as taught by the physiotherapist.

● Discreet raisers found for the settee.

● The parents were delighted to have a plan that may help with transfers in the living room and away from home.

Assessment review data six months later

Sophie preferred the handler completing the front transfer as it was easier for her

Time to complete: **2-5** minutes

Handler Effort **6** (although physically now easier, the task requires more mental effort and more encouragement to be given)

Risk to Sophie **Low.**

* Data in red indicates changes.

2 Transfers from posture seating to wheelchair

Example: at an after-school club

Environment: large hall in a school used for an after-school club for children aged 5-11. Only one child who uses a wheelchair. Activities are set up in the hall, including games, painting, sports and floor activities.

Jed spends all afternoon in his specialised seating, which is difficult to move around, and is transferred into his powered wheelchair using a hoist in the hygiene room at end of session.

Although the hall is large, there are a lot of activities and the ability to move around in a powered wheelchair is complicated by safety issues.

The powered wheelchair is used to its fullest and is in poor repair: the single wide footplate does not stay upright when raised, the seat padding has deteriorated, and the side supports are damaged and loose.

A wheelchair assessment has been completed, but is unlikely to be approved within the next two months.

Task: after-school club staff lift Jed out of his powered chair onto the floor by supporting him under his arms (one person each side) and lowering him to the floor. He is lifted back into his powered chair at the end of the session by reversing the technique.

He is unable to stand, but has often been held upright for transfers as he has limited movement in his hips and knees and therefore does not sag if a person holds him.

Jed enjoys being hoisted, but becomes very upset if lowered onto the floor in front of friends.

He has also been complaining recently of pain under his arms, which the manual handling practitioner attributes to the lift in and out of the chair. His hip and knee flexion deformities are increasing as he is spending less and less time out of his chair.

Some staff at the club also work with Jed in school, but others are employed separately for the club. They have not had any manual handling training and therefore do not want to transfer Jed onto/off the floor. The school staff are not always available to help, and have refused to lift Jed to the floor as they feel it is high risk.

Issues: it is not advisable for Jed to remain in his powered chair for the duration of the club, especially as there are a number of activities he could take part in that would help prevent further deterioration of his hip and knee movement range.

The wheelchair needs repair or replacement.

Lifting a person on/off the floor is difficult to complete in a controlled and safe way.

Options Investigated

● Raiser cushion

● Training of After School Staff in backcare and manual handling (including hoists).

● Trial of alternative method (using a stable chair for Jed to lean on in front of two people (one either side) while a third person removes the powered wheelchair – and Jed eases himself to the floor – reversing the method to get him back into the chair.

● Review wheelchair assessment to consider powered version which lowers to the floor, so that Jed can crawl in and out by himself or be assisted with slide sheets.

● Bringing him into the hall first (if possible) and hoisting him to the floor before his friends arrive.

Outcome

● Jed used the three-person technique initially, but using three handlers was not viable.

● When possible the hoist was used for some transfers.

● The wheelchair specification was changed and a new chair (which lowered to the floor) arrived six months after the assessment.

Child ability	3

Child size: D
Child comfort: 2
Child risk: Medium

BEFORE

Handler effort: **15**
Risk to handler: **high**

* Competent handler assessed as required

Child ability	3

Child size: D
Child comfort: 7
Child risk: Low

AT SIX MONTH REVIEW

* Data in red indicates changes

Handler effort: **10**
Risk to handler: **medium**
Time to complete: **2-5 mins**
Handler skill: **Ab**

3 Helping child on play equipment

Lifting child on/off a swing and onto the first rung of a climbing frame, and helping them down again.

Environment: an outdoor play area, with swings and climbing frames. The matting has been designed to avoid injury to a falling child. The weather is variable, but the play area is unlikely to be used in the rain or extreme weather.

Sam has a genetic disorder which means he has a poor sense of danger. He has fixed flexion deformities at his knees, and wears a caliper on his shortened right leg. He needs to be very active and has a lot of energy.

If he spends too much time sitting still he starts to self harm and become distressed.

He is able to stand, walk and run, but easily trips. Sam mostly runs, and staff have been unable to encourage him to slow down. He has much more energy than all the staff, and is either running around or quickly falling asleep.

He tends to become very attached to one person and will not respond to anyone else while that person is available. Sam also tends to grab and pull the person working with him. He laughs and continues the activity if he thinks he has hurt someone or if they attempt to tell him to stop doing something that is dangerous.

Staff allocated to work with Sam tend to be young, new people as they are perceived as more likely to be fit, but even they are quickly becoming exhausted.

Josie (new member of staff) has requested a transfer to work with other children as she is experiencing exhaustion and back ache after a 30 minute session with Sam.

Issues

Sam's safety while on the equipment.

The frustration of those working with Sam – they feel there are no options to improve the situation.

Sam's need to be very active and his lack of a sense of danger

Length of time staff are running around with him.

Options Investigated

● Introduction of a behaviour management programme, in conjunction with learning more about Sam and how he views the world.

● Swapping staff every 10 minutes.

● Investigating safer areas for Sam to play (soft play areas/ball pool).

● Training for staff on human movement and principles of moving and handling, in order that that they are more pro-active when assisting Sam on and off equipment.

● Requesting funding for more suitable equipment for children such as Sam.

Outcome

■ The behaviour management programme gave staff a strategy to follow, leading to reduced frustration.

■ Swapping staff was successful, providing the person who had previously been with Sam was in a completely different area.

■ Using soft play facilities was a success, Sam enjoyed such facilities much more than the outdoor equipment.

Child ability	5

Child size:	F	
Child comfort:	6	**BEFORE**
Child risk:	high	

Handler effort:	**20**
Risk to handler:	**very high**

Child ability	5

Handler skill level has risen from Novice to Competent.

Child size:	F	
Child comfort:	9	*AT SIX*
Child risk:	low	*MONTH*
		REVIEW

Handler effort:	**14**
Risk to handler:	**medium**

* Data in red indicates changes

And finally...

This book cannot deal with all the problems which may be encountered when working with mobility impaired children and young people. However, it may provide guidance in the use of a problem solving approach.

A risk benefit analysis will inform handlers of potential evidence-based benefits of the proposed action, contrasted with its potential risks. This should allow them to make informed decisions as to any amendments that are necessary for its safe performance. Physiotherapists, occupational therapists and manual handling practitioners can all offer advice on manual handling matters, but the employer of handlers carrying them out must be aware of the risks involved, and provide suitable training to enable their workforce to work safely.

It is always better to plan for the future when designing/equipping a building for use by people with special needs. Retro-fitting is often more expensive, less satisfactory and likely to limit potential for future changes. Involving professionals, as well as those who are to work in the setting, should enable a suitable environment to be provided for children which is ergonomically designed for all users, including families, handlers, and volunteers ■

Personal care

This section considers the moving and handling options available for assisting a child with personal care, from assisting with toileting to bathing. Much of the following information is equally applicable to children of both genders.

It is important to consider any intimate care policies of the organisations involved.

✱ ***Even though only one person may be required for the technique, there may be an intimate care policy requirement – to protect children and staff – that two people are present.***

1 Helping standing child change a pad

Some children prefer to be assisted with personal care such as changing a pad or nappy while standing.

The child usually stands holding a bar or by the side of a stable change table. Sometimes, if the child is small and their wheelchair high, a step can help.

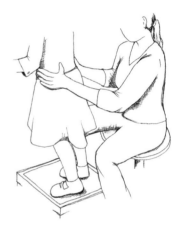

Child ability	5 - 7

Child size: **B - E**

Child comfort: **10**

 Wheelie stool, seat or kneeler pad, step (appropriate height for child), bar or surface for child to hold, and relevant protective equipment for handler.

Handler effort: **6 - 9**

Risk to handler: **medium**

(shoulders & lower back)

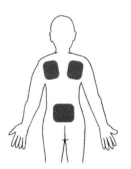

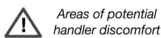 *Areas of potential handler discomfort*

Considerations: behaviour patterns of the child, ability of the child to reliably weightbear, suitability of equipment which is used for support, space, type of pad or nappy used.

Alternatives: no alternatives are easily suggested, unless the child is unsteady and could then benefit from use of a standing harness for support in standing.

If a child is able to partially weightbear (but NOT when they are known to suddenly drop) they can lean forward onto a changing bed, with the second person giving some support.

If a child requires a great deal of assistance to stand, they could lie on a change table, which is adjusted to their height for the transfer. Handler then raises table to suitable height for working. Child may be able to 'bridge' or lift their bottom off the surface to help with clothing etc.

2 Helping standing child use urine bottle

The handler sits on a stool of appropriate height, supporting the child from behind.

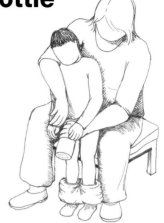

Child ability **5 - 7**

Child size: **C**

Child comfort: **10**

 Wheelie stool, seat or kneeler pad, step (appropriate height for child), fixed bar for child to use for support, urinal and relevant protective equipment for handler.

Handler effort: **6 - 9**

Risk to handler: **low**

(shoulders & lower back)

Considerations: wheelie stool or seat may help avoid stooped posture or kneeling by handler, bar can be fixed to a wall for child to use as support. The behaviour patterns of the child, their ability to reliably weightbear and suitability of support equipment will all have a bearing on the task.

Alternatives: using the bottle or female urinal in a sitting position may be possible for some children.

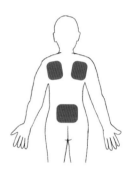

 Areas of potential handler discomfort

3 Helping child in chair use urine bottle

Child may need guidance to adjust their position in the chair, and help with clothing in order to use a urine bottle or female urinal while seated.

Child ability **3 - 5**

Child size: **D - F**

Child comfort: **8 - 10**

 Urinal and relevant protective equipment for handler.

Handler effort: **6 - 15**

Depending on child's weight, ability & muscle tone.

Risk to handler: **low**

Providing handlers do not attempt to lift child (shoulders, upper & lower back)

Considerations: child's behaviour patterns, ability to assist, weight, physical disabilities; wheelchair controls, eg does it have tilt facility/ height adjustment which can help handler assisting good posture and avoid over-exertion. Child usually needs loose fitting trousers for this option. Sometimes hoist required as child is not able to wriggle backwards and forwards in chair.

Alternatives: hoist and sling, using urine bottle while briefly suspended safely in hoist, one-way glide sheets to help child back in the seat.

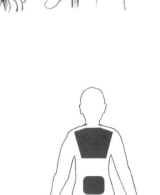

 Areas of potential handler discomfort

4 Using transfer board to swap seats

The area is prepared and is preferably of equal height to the wheelchair, an arm of which is removed and the sliding board inserted. Child slides along board to the receiving seat, often holding on to arm of chair for support. This transfer is usually used where child has good upper body strength but cannot stand. It can be used in the hygiene room, classroom or anywhere which has seating of very similar height to child's wheelchair.

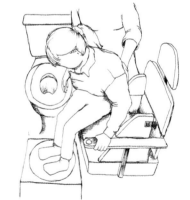

 Child ability 5 - 7

Child size: **D - F**
Child comfort: **10**

 Transfer board. Suitable height, or height adjustable, seating.

  ↑A^b 1-2

Handler effort: **6**
Risk to handler: **low**
(supervisory role only)

⚠ *No handler discomfort issues in supervisory role*

Considerations: child must be able to support their own head and upper body, be confident in reaching for chair and not feel that they may fall. Ensure child does not place hands over transfer board edge as there is risk of trapping fingers.

Handler may be tempted to consider using handling belt to pull child along, but this significantly increases risk of injury to themselves, impedes child's independence and also places child at higher risk of falling.

Alternatives: use of board with attached slide sheet to allow easier movement – but this requires detailed risk assessment, due to risk of child slipping off.

5 Toilet transfer with portable raised step

Used where child's feet do not reach the ground but independent transfer needs to be encouraged. Child will only be taking a small amount of weight on their feet, mostly using their hands to help with the transfer.

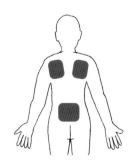

Child ability 5 - 6

Child size: **B - D**
Child comfort: **8 - 10**

 Raised block with turndisc if suitable. Rails fixed to the toilet, or very close to it, and accessible for the child.

 * ↑C 1-2

Handler effort: **6**
Risk to handler: **low**
(shoulders & lower back)

Considerations: child needs good upper-body strength for this transfer. Handler must not be tempted to lift. A second person, if present, stands in front to ensure child is safe. Clothing removed once child over the toilet.

Alternatives: hoist and access sling, powered stand aid depending on size of child.

 ⚠ *Areas of potential handler discomfort*

6 Hoisting child from chair to toilet using sling

Child is hoisted using an access sling which means clothing can be removed, while they are in the sling, without taking them out of the sling. Some-upper body control is usually needed (see equipment section and notes below).

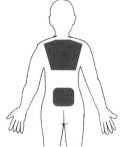

Child ability **3 - 5**

Child size: **All**
Child comfort: **10**

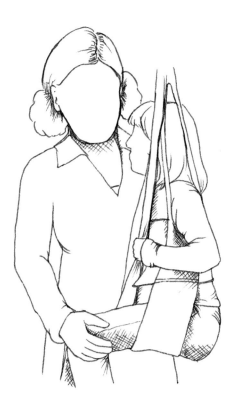

Hoist and access sling, male or female urinal and relevant protective equipment for handler.

Handler effort: **6 - 15**
Risk to handler: **low**
(depending on weight, muscle tone and ability of child)

⚠ *Areas of potential handler discomfort*

Considerations: child's behaviour patterns, their ability to assist, weight and physical disabilities, and the type of sling may determine whether they can be hoisted directly onto the toilet.

For standard access slings child, while in sitting position, must be able to reliably control their head and trunk and keep their arms outside the of sling.

Different access slings include those which can be used when child has less head and trunk control.

● An individual assessment by a competent person must be completed prior to selecting appropriate method.

Special techniques can be taught to assist handler in helping replace trousers without having to remove sling.

Alternatives: hoist and toileting sling which doesn't rely on hook and loop fasteners but uses a strap providing compression around the chest. Hoist and universal sling. Transfer to toilet after first removing clothing on a change table, which will require more time.

7 Helping child in sling use urine bottle

Child uses urine bottle while supported in a hoist and sling. Picture shows wishbone-type spreader bar which may give better access. This is sometimes used with the sling leg-pieces uncrossed for a 2 point spreader bar. Child is raised out of chair, remaining slightly above seat. This method is sometimes used for boys who are unable to stand and cannot use a bottle while sitting in chair.

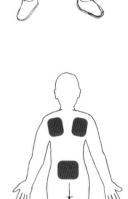

Child ability 2 - 4	Child size: D - F
	Child comfort: 8 - 10

 Hoist, appropriate sling, male or female urinal, relevant protective equipment for handler.

Handler effort: **10 - 12**
Risk to handler: **medium**
(shoulders & lower back)

● Competent person required to assess safety of using adapted sling.

Considerations: ability of child to be safely supported in sling with uncrossed leg pieces, agreement from the hoist/sling company that sling can be used with uncrossed leg pieces, ease of clothing removal (loose trousers/adapted clothing usually needed for this).

Alternatives: Investigation of alternative slings/options for passing urine, eg some children have intermittent catheterisation.

 Areas of potential handler discomfort

8 Lifting child to changing table

Manually lifting small child onto change table by supporting them around the lower chest. A baby or more dependent child would require more support from handler.

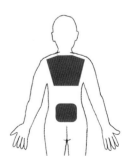

Child ability 1 - 7	Child size: A - B
	Child comfort: 8 - 10

 Change bed – preferably height adjustable.

Handler effort: **6 - 15**
Risk to handler: **medium/high**
(shoulders & lower back)

Considerations: child's behaviour patterns, ability to assist, weight and physical disabilities. Space around change table (access to one side only will make task much more difficult). Sometimes a manual lift is performed with a child who is independent because of fixed-height table. Assessment/consideration of introducing height adjustable table. Provide step/steps/step-and-rails suitable to child.

Alternatives: hoist and sling. Two person lift (only following specific individual assessment, and probably as interim measure).

 Areas of potential handler discomfort

9 Two people lifting child to change table

Manually lifting a child onto a change table, one person lifting around the torso, and another person lifting legs.

Child ability **2 - 5**

Child size: **B - C**
Child comfort: **5 - 7**

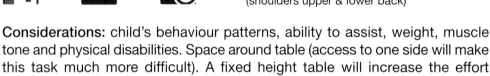

 Change bed (preferably height adjustable).

Handler effort: **9 - 15**
Risk to handler: **medium**
(shoulders upper & lower back)

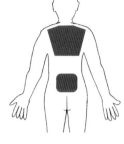

Considerations: child's behaviour patterns, ability to assist, weight, muscle tone and physical disabilities. Space around table (access to one side will make this task much more difficult). A fixed height table will increase the effort required and risk level.

Alternatives: hoist and sling, adjusting technique so that handler lifting torso avoids holding forearms (only possible with very light children with good shoulder control). Enough space to take one step between the chair and table, practising to improve posture. Second handler supporting closer to the child's hips rather than their knees.

 Areas of potential handler discomfort

● This technique is often uncomfortable for child, and may make them feel they are slipping.

10 Hoisting child to change table

Showering/bathing: the many different options for bathing depend on child's size, health, ability to help and the space, funding and availability of help. Specific assessment is needed for each situation. Examples listed are common scenarios in schools or aqua-therapy pools in special schools. Contact occupational therapist for specific advice.

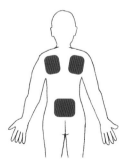

Child ability **1 - 4**

Child size: **B - F**
Child comfort: **8 - 10**

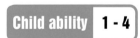

 Hoist, sling, change bed, relevant handler protection equipment.

Handler effort: **11 - 15**
Risk to handler: **medium**
(shoulders & lower back)

Considerations: two people may be needed depending on child's, size, behaviour patterns, ability to assist and physical disabilities. Space around table (access to only one side will make task much more difficult). Slide sheets can be used for positioning. Positioning sheets/turning devices used with hoist may also help.

Alternatives: this is usually the lower risk method of assisting a child onto table for personal care.

Areas of potential handler discomfort

11 Showering child on pull down seat

Child sits on shower seat or shower chair and may have been able to complete a standing transfer, or may have been hoisted onto seat. There are many different types of seat and an occupational therapist will be able to help in assessment and selection of the most appropriate.

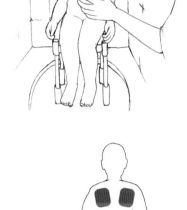

Child ability **5 - 7**

Child size: **C - F**

Child comfort: **9**

 Shower, seat, protective clothing for handler.

Handler effort: **11 - 13**

Risk to handler: **low**

(shoulders & lower back)

Considerations: ability of child to sit on drop down seat, height of drop down seat from the handlers' perspective, space required around child, air temperature, availability of grab-rails for additional support.

Alternatives: specialised shower chair, shower trolley or specialist height-adjustable bath with supportive inserts.

Areas of potential handler discomfort

12 Showering on wheeled shower-seat or commode

Child is hoisted or manually lifted into shower chair and straps secured, as required. Chair then pushed into level access shower area and assistant washes child.

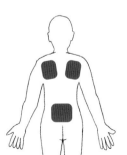

Child ability **1 - 2**

Child size: **B - F**

Child comfort: **9**

 Appropriate wheeled shower-seat, protective equipment for handlers, hoist and sling.

Handler effort: **6**

Risk to handler: **low**

(shoulders & lower back)

Considerations: level access to shower area required enabling wheeled shower-chair to be pushed into shower if required. Child may need chair reclined to assist postural control, and to be secured by straps.

Alternatives: shower trolley, special supportive seat in bath (mainly for smaller children).

● Two handlers for hoisting as child requires careful positioning in seat.

Areas of potential handler discomfort

13 Showering child on shower-trolley

Trolley has padded base and sides. It is usually tillted slightly downwards towards drain at bottom, which is channelled to sink/drain. Child is hoisted or manually lifted onto trolley. Technique useful for children without ability to sit.

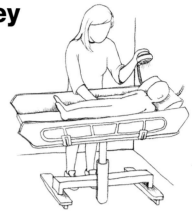

Child ability **1 - 4**

Child size: **B - F**

Child comfort: **9**

Shower trolley, shower, protective equipment for handlers, hoist and sling for transfer.

Handler effort: **8**

Risk to handler: **low**

(shoulders & lower back)

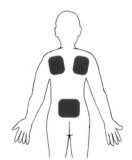

Considerations: air temperature, width of shower trolley, remembering to raise shower trolley to avoid stooping.

Alternatives: whole-body wash in bed, inflatable bath with drain which can be used on bed, height adjustable bath with suitable inserts.

 Areas of potential handler discomfort

---

14 Helping child to roll

Task spans many activities (placing sling, showering, personal care, dressing, applying body braces). Child is supported and rolled. Roll should (usually) be towards handler – not away – to avoid over-reaching. Handler should aim to support child's shoulder and hip to avoid child's discomfort.

Child ability **1 - 4**

Child size: **B - F**

Child comfort: **9**

Height adjustable surface with side rails.

Handler effort: **8 - 20**

Risk to handler: **low**

(shoulders & lower back)

Considerations: width of surface, size, weight and ability of child. Task may be very easy in ideal circumstances with small child, but is increasingly harder if child is less able, heavier, and the surface narrow. Be aware of increased difficulties or discomfort if child has unstable hips, a body brace or a body shape making it difficult for them to turn.

If slide sheets are used to aid roll, child's back will be towards handler, rather than their front. Tables fixed to wall may add to difficulties due to reduced access.

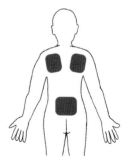

 Areas of potential handler discomfort

Transfers – standing & walking

In class or living rooms: many children need assistance with walking. Useful walking or standing ability will promote easier transfers for handlers.

Some may need only verbal prompting or a helping hand, while others require a standing harness and hoist.

An upright position is beneficial to most children, but assistance required to achieve this varies. Some need a walker with saddle to rest on when tired – which can be enjoyable, as they can often 'scoot' about quite fast!

Children unable to stand and walk may use a standing frame to encourage weightbearing and upright posture (covered in equipment section).

15 Helping from sitting to standing

Child is encouraged to stand by two handlers, one each side. It is expected that the handlers are supporting – not lifting. Child must have feet on the ground and be compliant. A handling belt may provide a better handhold for helpers.

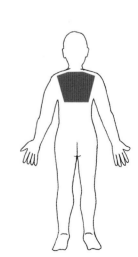

Child ability | **5 - 7**

Child size: **B - F**
Child comfort: **8 - 10**

 None.

Handler effort: **8 - 13**
Risk to handler: **medium**
(shoulders & upper back)

Considerations: predictability of child, weightbearing ability, height of seat.

Alternatives: Can be undertaken by one handler, if child can help sufficiently. Stand and turn aid, standing harness and hoist.

⚠ *Areas of potential handler discomfort*

16 Sit to stand from front

For child with visual impairment (with additional help from side if necessary). Child encouraged to stand using a person in front. It is not expected that handler will take any weight, but simply provide a visual/sensory cue to child, who must be compliant.

 Child ability 5 - 7

Child size: C - F
Child comfort: 8 - 10

None.

Handler effort: **8 - 13**
Risk to handler: **low**
(shoulders & upper back)

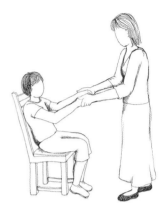

Considerations: technique should not be used to pull child out of chair – this could damage their shoulders and the handler's back. A second person can be used to guide child's hips and to support first handler. Method can place handler at high risk if child does not move forward at the right time, or pulls backwards. Although it is often used because children tend to feel safer with a handler in front, it is not often recommended by manual handling practitioners.

Alternatives: two handlers, either one to remain at front with second at side supporting the pelvis or key points (if the handler has received training on key points) or use two handlers – one each side – to offer more support.

Consider walking harness to encourage child to push up from the seat for a more usual sit to stand process.

If child is only standing (not preparing to walk) some handlers sit and allow child to place hands on their forearms, for steadying only, with second handler supporting at side. Proceed with caution if child is large, unreliable or unsteady.

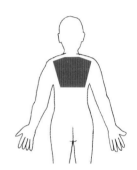

Areas of potential handler discomfort

17 Helping to walk with wheelie stool

Handler sits on adjustable wheelie stool, supporting child around trunk or by key point of control on top of shoulder (where the handler has been instructed specifically in using key points) with child facing either forwards or backwards.

 Child ability 5 - 6

Child size: B - C
Child comfort: 8

 Wheelie stool.

Handler effort: **12**
Risk to handler: **low**
(shoulders & lower back)

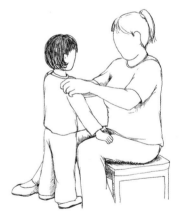

Considerations: handler assisting should only do so for as long as they are comfortable, and should stop for regular rests. There is a tendency to continue too long and feel uncomfortable later.

Continued on opposite page

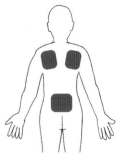

Areas of potential handler discomfort

Continued from previous page

Ensure wheelie stool is set at correct height for handler so they do not need to stoop.

This method is also dependent on co-operation, predictability and compliance of child. Not all wheelie stools are suitable for this task. 'Star'-based types, with small swivel tops, are unlikely to tip and may allow the handler to keep close.

If rectangular seat type is used, it is important that handler sits astride seat to achieve the greatest stability.

18 Helping child walk with walking frame

Child walks supported by walking frame, which is often used behind them to facilitate access to activities in front of them.

Child ability 4 - 6

Child size: B - F
Child comfort: 8

 Walking frame.

Handler effort: **10**
Risk to handler: **low**
(lower back)

Considerations: Child must have some weight bearing ability and be able to reliably hold onto frame. Child may need help from second person, or a chair brought up behind them when about to sit if they find turning difficult.

Alternatives: child could be hoisted into more supportive walking frame, perhaps with a central saddle.

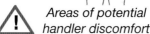

Areas of potential handler discomfort

19 Stand and turn aid

Used for children able to partially or fully weightbear, but have difficulty turning their feet. Child places feet on the device and pulls on handles to stand. Once child is upright, handler will turn wheeled turner before child then lowers onto new seat.

Child ability 5 - 7

Child size: C - F
Child comfort: 8 - 10

 Standing and turning device, handle must be low enough for child to reach.

Handler effort: **8 - 13**
Risk to handler: **low**
(shoulders & lower back)

Considerations: different equipment manufacturers have different designs. Some require two handlers and others one. Training and advice is needed to ensure appropriate method and number of people are used, which will also depend on task being performed (simple turn or as part of toileting). This equipment should not be used to help child up from floor.

Alternatives: turning disc and two assistants, standing harness and hoist, powered stand aid, powered assistive standing frame – if these are suitable to size of child.

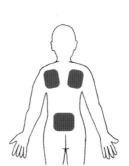

 Areas of potential handler discomfort

20 Helping child to walk with walking harness

Child, supported by walking harness on mobile hoist/tracking, is encouraged to walk by handler who may sit on wheeled stool if child is small.

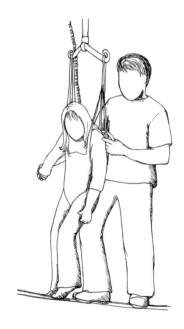

Child ability 3 - 4

Child size: B - F
Child comfort: 8

 Overhead tracking hoist or hoist that works in a similar way, with a short spreader bar as required, and walking harness.

Handler effort: **10**
Risk to handler: **low**
(lower back)

Considerations: child must have some weightbearing ability. If using tracking be aware of spreader bar spinning, causing sensory difficulties for child and risk of handler being hit on head with spreader bar.

Also: child's predictability, understanding and co-operation. Two people required if using mobile hoist (one to push hoist).

Alternatives: child could be hoisted into walker.

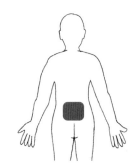

 Areas of potential handler discomfort

Floor work

Many children with impaired mobility are able to get about on the floor by crawling or rolling.

This sense of freedom is often an important part of their day. However many adults are not comfortable on the floor, or have difficulties in getting back up.

Many exercise regimes are undertaken on the floor, and these may often be made safer for the handler by performing them on a height-adjustable couch.

Sitting with a pillow between calves and thighs, or using a 'meditation' stool may allow adults more comfort on the floor.

21 Off floor (independent)

Area is prepared – wheelchair brakes are placed ON – and child uses the chair to move from floor into the seat (or perhaps a classroom chair). This is usually by child adopting a half-kneeling position before pushing on the chair to stand, but sometimes they can lift themselves directly back into the chair from the floor if they have strong arm muscles and chair is not too high.

Child ability	5 - 7

Child size: **C - F**
Child comfort: **8 - 10**

 None.

 ↑N

 Handler effort: **6**
Risk to handler: **low**

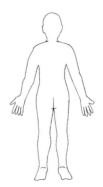

Considerations: transfer may be more difficult if child has splints in their shoes as this reduces the amount of movement of their ankles.
Child also has to be able to co-ordinate their movements. Ensure wheelchair footplates are removed or pushed back to the side. Any chair may need to be stabilised as the child is getting up.

Alternatives: try an inflatable raiser cushion or hoist and sling.

 No issues

22 Transfer between floor and low seat

This technique is useful if handler can support child in standing position. Child uses arms of chair to take some of their weight and moves around to gradually step and turn prior to sitting back in seat. They may need footplates replaced before pushing back into seat. Some can climb into wheelchair, but only if is suitable and brakes are firmly on.

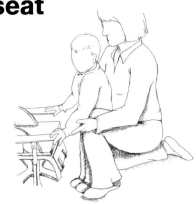

Child ability 4 - 5

Child size: A - B
Child comfort: 8

 None.

Handler effort: **10**
Risk to handler: **low**
(shoulders, spine, knees & ankles)

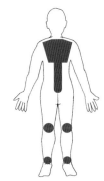

Considerations: handler's ability of handler to kneel and balance, child's height, weight, ability to partially weightbear and follow instructions.

Alternatives: standing harness, hoist and sling if the child is unreliable.

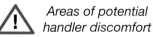 *Areas of potential handler discomfort*

23 Helping child on handler's lap to stand

Handler kneels back on heels, draws child onto lap (a slide sheet may help) then, supporting child at hips and remaining close, rises to kneeling up high, with child standing, often with child pulling on rail to assist.

Child ability 3 - 5

Child size: A - B
Child comfort: 8 - 10

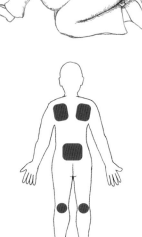

 Usually use a ladder back chair, or grab-rails on wall.

Handler effort: **9**
Risk to handler: **medium**
(shoulders, upper, lower back, knees)

Considerations: care should be taken if child is not holding onto bar etc in front, as if they lose balance they may pull handler over. If child is tall it will be harder for their movements to be controlled by the handler.

Alternatives: sit to stand with standing harness and hoist.

 Areas of potential handler discomfort

24 Using inflatable raiser cushion to/from floor

Child is usually able to push themselves or to be rolled onto a flat cushion, following the manufacturer's instructions. Slide sheets can sometimes be used. One person supports child as cushion is inflated one cell at a time (up to 4 cells). Number of cells inflated depends on height of child, who will usually stand to transfer once everyone is ready

Child ability 4 - 6

Child size: C - F
Child comfort: 8 - 10

 Raiser cushion and compressor. Some children benefit from using slide sheets to get onto cushion.

Handler effort: **8 - 11**
Risk to handler: **low**
(knees, ankles, hips)

Considerations: child needs some trunk stability, must not be startled by noises from compressor (or at least be able to manage once told). To maintain stability child must be reminded to move their feet back as cushion inflates. Cushion can be used to lower child to floor, although this is not its primary function. The manufacturer's instructions must always be followed.

Alternatives: hoist and whole body sling

 Areas of potential handler discomfort

25 Floor to-from buggy, corner or low seat

Kneeling or crouching to lift small child using a scoop lift, from the side, to transfer into a low seat

Child ability 1 - 2

Child size: A - B
Child comfort: 8

 Low seat for child

Handler effort: **10**
Risk to handler: **medium**
(shoulders, lower back, hips, knees & ankles)

Considerations: Ability of handler to kneel or squat, child's weight and particular health needs. Brakes should always be on any wheeled seat. Task may be harder if the buggy has sloped seat or non-removable foot support. May be possible to complete task in the kneeling position if equipment is easily accessible, but care must be taken as lifting ability is reduced in that position. If lifting into a corner seat, it is harder to keep close to the child as they are lowered into it, and second person may be required to clear area or arrange equipment.

Alternatives: passing technique (if it is necessary to stand up while holding child), hoist and appropriate sling, corner seat with removable pommel so child can crawl into position rather than being lifted over pommel.

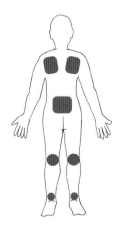

 Areas of potential handler discomfort

26 Hoisting child to-from floor

Mobile hoist or overhead tracking is used to lift child from chair or bed to floor with standard sling positioned around the child.

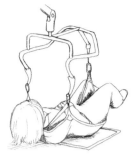

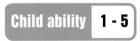 **1 - 5**

Child size: **B - F**

Child comfort: **6 - 9**

 Mobile hoist or overhead tracking (preferably H frame), slide sheets if using a mobile hoist.

Handler effort: **8 - 11**

Risk to handler: **low**

(knees & lower back)

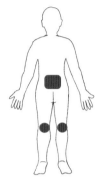

Considerations: one handler may be able to complete task, but detailed consideration of particular circumstances (staff ability to work on floor, space/busyness of the area) would be needed. Careful planning required, if using mobile hoist, re which direction child is approached.

If using slide sheets, it is possible with many hoists to approach child from their head end, thus avoiding lifting, moving or trying to move hoist around child's legs (check with manufacturer). Place slide sheet under child's bottom at same time as sling.

Be aware some children with unpredictable movements or increased tone may not tolerate slippery feeling of being on slide sheet. Sheet must not protrude into working area (risk of helpers slipping). For children with involuntary movements, care must be taken to prevent contact with hoist frame.

Areas of potential handler discomfort

Alternatives: working on raised wide bench, rather than floor.

27 Manual lift of small child from low surface

Lifting small child from low surface with child held facing handler. If child has extensor spasms, they may be held with back to handler. Handler, stands from half-kneeling position.

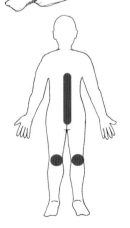

 1

Child size: **A - B**

Child comfort: **8**

 None.

Handler effort: **9**

Risk to handler: **medium**

(lumbar spine, knees)

Considerations: handler's ability to kneel, and to stand from that position while holding child. Child's weight and muscle tone, and whether they startle easily.

Alternatives: passing technique (to a handler or into a seat), slide onto handler's lap cradling head and legs before standing, hoist and sling, lifting sling (which would require two handlers).

 Areas of potential handler discomfort

28 Lifting from floor with lifting sling

Lifting sling (very similar to a hoisting sling) is placed around the small child and they are lifted using the handles and keeping close. Either the wheelchair is directly behind the staff and the child (with the brakes on) or a third person could bring in the chair.

Technique is useful for introducing child to slings, particularly in nursery or confined areas, as it does not take up as much room as a mobile hoist.

Care must be taken that this is not used with larger children, for whom it should be considered as an interim or emergency technique only.

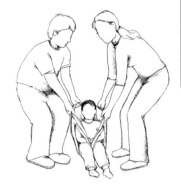

Child ability 1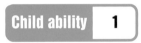

Child size: A - B
Child comfort: 8

 Lifting sling.

Handler effort: **12**
Risk to handler: **medium**
(lumbar spine & knees)

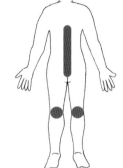

Considerations: handler's ability to stand/reach in this position holding the child. Child's weight and muscle tone and whether they startle easily or have extensor spasms. At least one handler will need to work on the floor to place the sling, and possibly to support child from behind.

 Areas of potential handler discomfort

Alternatives: hoist and sling.

Therapy, pools, play and riding

Leisure, therapy and recreation can often be combined by using suitable play activities.

Most children enjoy using a ball – and swimming and riding can give them a sense of independence, as well as being fun and enabling social interaction with their peers.

Ball pools may cause access problems for mobile hoists, unless there is room for the hoist base beneath the pool (raised supports providing clearance). Tracking or a gantry over the pool can give easier access.

Standing Frame Transfers: therapists often prescribe a 'standing' regime for *children unable to stand unaided. This helps retain their joint movement range and muscle length, and may increase bone density.*

Facilitating head control, it aims to improve abnormal muscle tone and allows them to work at a table with other children. It also provides a different perspective on their surroundings and allows peer interaction with standing children.

However, helping a child into and out of this equipment may prove problematic for handlers. Therapists must ensure that the handlers involved have an appropriate skill level.

29 Assisting child into stander from bed

Transferring partially weightbearing child into prone or upright stander from change bed. Child is perched on edge of change table with their feet placed into the foot plate on the standing frame. One handler either side guides child into standing position and fixes pelvic band, followed by the chest band and all other straps, unless written otherwise according to circumstances.

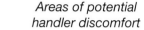

Child ability	3 - 7

Child size: C - E
Child comfort: 6 - 9

 Standing frame, height adjustable change table.

Handler effort: **6 - 15**
Risk to handler: **medium/high**
(shoulders & lower back)

Areas of potential handler discomfort

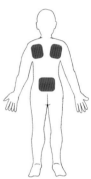

Considerations: method should not be used for unpredictable child who experiences muscle spasms causing their position to change rapidly, or who has feet fixed by orthoses or calipers, or if they cannot assist sufficiently.

Alternatives: standing harness with overhead tracking/mobile hoist, or a supine stander. Variations on standing frames include self-propelled wheeled versions, specialist walking frames, walking harnesses – either off-the-peg types or specialist items such as a neoprene harness – can be used.

30 Transferring seated child into upright stander

Technique used for children who can assist and are at least partially weightbearing. The stander is brought in front of child, who is usually seated in chair, with one handler standing either side. Child places feet into foot plates on standing frame. Handling belt can be used to assist standing up, but must NOT be used to lift child. Once child is in frame, the hip strap is usually positioned first.

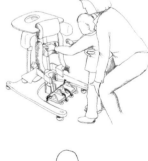

Child ability	1

Child size: B - F
Child comfort: 8

 Standing frame (handling belt (where appropriate).

Handler effort: **12**
Risk to handler: **medium/high**
(lumbar spine, knees & shoulders)

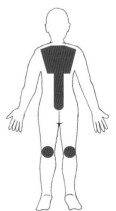

Considerations: weightbearing ability of child is the most important factor. Unreliable or unpredictable children can easily slip, putting themselves and handlers at risk. A physiotherapist will usually be very involved with therapy programme for this equipment, and should be consulted for individual advice on access and positioning.

 Areas of potential handler discomfort

Continued on opposite page

Continued from previous page

Alternatives: hoist and standing harness, tilt standing frame, child can sit on or be hoisted onto handler's knee behind standing frame (providing both feel comfortable and that child assists in the stand). Child's feet placed on footplates by other handler and both handlers guide child up into standing. For more able children this can also be achieved by them sitting on end of a changing plinth which is gradually raised until they are almost standing (see task 29).

31 Hoisting child into prone standing frame

Standing harness is usually placed on child while they sit in wheelchair. Once child is hoisted into upright position, the wheelchair is removed and they may be secured in the stander. They may also be gently turned through 180 degrees to face the prone standing frame, if hoisted from in front.

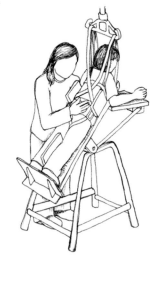

Child is raised sufficiently in hoist to clear footplates of the stander. Supporting straps are placed around child while they are still supported in sling.

Once child is secure, tension in the sling is reduced by slightly lowering hoist and the straps removed from hoist. The harness is usually left in situ, as it can be difficult to remove/replace in the stander.

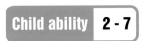 **Child ability** 2 - 7

Child size: C - F
Child comfort: 6 - 10

 Prone standing frame, standing harness, overhead tracking (preferred) or suitable hoist to fit round standing frame and which has sufficient lift height.

Handler effort: **9**
Risk to handler: **low**
(shoulders, lower back)

Considerations: although standing harness avoids physically lifting child into position, handlers often still stoop to strap the feet.

It is also important to secure hip band early otherwise child may slide down and feel increased discomfort under their arms, or even feel their airway is restricted.

Sling may be uncomfortable for the student if left in place, however, it is not feasible to remove and replace while child is in the frame. Standing harnesses are not always suitable for students with feeding PEGS.

Alternatives: supine standing frame with whole body sling and overhead tracking hoist or mobile hoist (tracking hoist preferable).

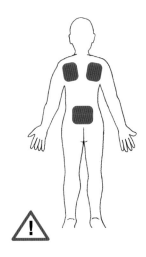

Areas of potential handler discomfort

32 Hoisting to supine standing frame or tilt table

Standard sling is placed on child in their chair or a change bed. Child is hoisted onto flat supine standing frame or table. Sling is tucked out of the way or removed. Straps are secured to support child and usually include the feet, knees, hips and chest. Stander is then tilted to appropriate angle.

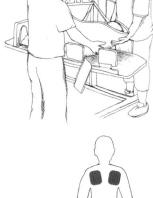

Child ability 1 - 5

Child size: B - F
Child comfort: 8 - 10

 Supine stander, hoist with enough clearance to lift to the horizontal tilt table, or overhead tracking.

Handler effort: **12**
Risk to handler: **low**
(shoulders & lower back)

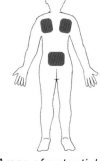

Considerations: handlers need to know how supine stander works, what adjustments can be made, what is removable, and how straps secure child. Slide sheets may help with positioning on some tilt tables.

Alternatives: standing frame which starts as a chair, walking harness, prone stander, wheelchair which can come into standing.

⚠ *Areas of potential handler discomfort*

33 Hoisting child to ball

Child is hoisted onto ball using suitable hoist, overhead tracking and sling – usually for therapy or play. Whether standing harness or standard sling are used will decide position of child on ball (eg sitting or on tummy).

Sling is left in situ with varying amounts of slack, depending on child's balance. As child progresses, sling can be replaced with an access sling or standing harness. Balance reactions can still be challenged but child is safe.

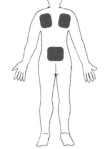

Child ability 2 - 5

Child size: B - F
Child comfort: 8 - 10

 Appropriate size ball, hoist and sling.

Handler effort: **12**
Risk to handler: **medium**
(shoulders & lower back)

Considerations: handler assisting should be confident with use of therapy balls, and would normally have been shown by physiotherapist; child's size, compliance and predictability movement patterns.

Alternatives: consider soft play therapy in a different setting such as soft play or sensory room.

⚠ *Areas of potential handler discomfort*

34 Manual transfer to or from ball

Child is supported on stool, bench or chair, one handler guides them from seat, while second handler prepares to receive the child over the ball. This could be used for chair to ball transfer – or the movement reversed to transfer to another chair if handlers are practised in that move.

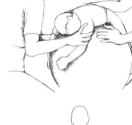

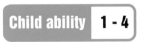 **Child ability 1 - 4**

Child size: A - C
Child comfort: 8 - 10

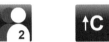

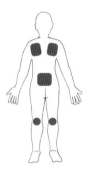

Handler effort: **11 - 16**
Risk to handler: **medium**
(shoulders, lower back & knees)

Considerations: handler's ability to move and support child. Child's health needs can affect task eg if they have sudden reflex movements or altering muscle tone. There is tendency to maintain stooped posture, therefore task must be regularly reviewed. Handlers can high kneel with cushioning under knees. Task will become more difficult as child grows.

Alternatives: use hoist and suitable sling, or discuss other therapy options with physiotherapist.

Areas of potential handler discomfort

35 Hoisting child to wedge

Standing harness used to lower child on their tummy onto a wedge. Neoprene harnesses usually work better for this. If able, and if appropriate, child can lower themselves using the remote control.

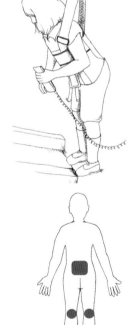

 Child ability 3 - 5

Child size: B - D
Child comfort: 6 - 8

 Low seat for child

Handler effort: **11**
Risk to handler: **low**
(lower back & knees)

Considerations: ensuring child's legs are not trapped if using mobile hoist Child may need some head control or an extra handler to support head. Depending on make of sling care needs to be taken regarding its straps, ensuring child is not caught or restricted. Encourage child to bend knees as they are lowered, to prevent a 'top heavy' posture placing additional pressure on their chest/shoulders.

Alternatives: Using standard hoist and sling onto inflatable wedge with child turned to face down, maybe using slide sheets to assist. Wedge then inflated.

 Areas of potential handler discomfort

63

36 Supported sitting

Small children spend a great deal of time on the floor at home and in early years education. There is often a desire by child, teacher and therapy staff that the child spends time on the floor with his or her peers, but they may not be able to support themselves in a sitting position. It is also a position used to maintain muscle length and joint range. The handler sits behind to offer support while child moves to and from floor using a method assessed as appropriate. Most adults will prefer to rest their backs against a firm support.

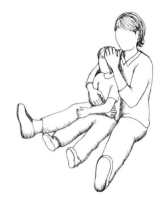

 Child ability **3 - 4**

Child size: **B - C**
Child comfort: **8 - 10**

 None.

Handler effort: **11 - 15**
Risk to handler: **medium**
(shoulders, lower back & arms)

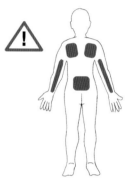

Considerations: child's behaviour patterns, ability to assist and physical disabilities; space, ability of handler to sit in long sitting. May be easier to lean against wall to avoid discomfort.

Alternatives: specialist floor seating (eg corner seat) to support child.

Areas of potential handler discomfort

37 Manually turning child to wedge or side-lier

Child may have been hoisted onto a wedge on floor but needs turning onto their tummy for therapy. Slide sheets are placed on wedge before child is hoisted onto it, and the top layer pulled to gently turn child. To avoid slipping, slide sheets may need 'locking' by a handler holding them in place while child is lowered onto wedge. If using side-lier, care must be taken that child does not roll off when turned, particularly if raised from floor.

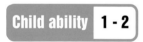 **Child ability** **1 - 2**

Child size: **B - D**
Child comfort: **8**

 Wedge, slide sheets of appropriate size.

Handler effort: **10**
Risk to handler: **medium**
(lumbar spine, knees & shoulders)

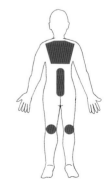

Considerations: ability of handler to kneel and rise unaided, child's weight and particular health needs, muscle tone, ability to roll; skill of handlers in using slide sheets. Some children find slide sheets difficult to cope with, and their use may increase muscle spasms.

Alternatives: using inflatable wedge so child can be rolled onto their tummy while the wedge is still flat, then inflating wedge. Sometimes specific walking harnesses can be used to eliminate need for turning, but require individual assessment. Height adjustable therapy beds are also available to replace fixed-height supportive equipment and/or need to work on floor.

Areas of potential handler discomfort

The swimming pool

38 Transferring small child to pool

Child is usually lifted from wheelchair or supportive shower chair to swimming/therapy pool edge, and passed to handler in pool. Usually only used for small children where pool has raised edge. Local procedures and guidance must be adhered to.

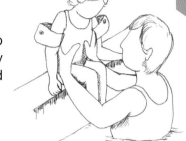

Child ability **3 - 5**

Child size: A - B
Child comfort: 8

 None

Handler effort: **12**
Risk to handler: **medium**
(spine, knees & shoulders)

Considerations: handler's ability to lift child from seat; weight and particular health needs of child, depth of pool, steps/slope, floor surface, wet environment/wet skin, water and atmospheric temperature.

Alternatives: pool hoist with seating or bed system, overhead tracking and sling. Some slings have floats attached to edges to aid application in water. Two handlers could also place child on flotation mat and slide them into water on it if pool sides and water surface are at floor level.

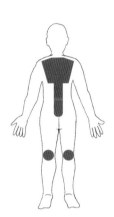

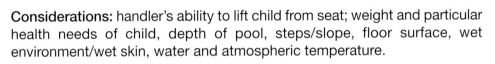 Areas of potential handler discomfort

39 Transfers using pool chair

Child completes standing transfer onto the seat or is hoisted onto it in change room. Chair is pushed to pool and attached to hoist with suitable straps providing child with some protection.

Child ability **4 - 7**

Child size: D - F
Child comfort: 9

 Pool hoist and chair.

Handler effort: **11**
Risk to handler: **low**
(shoulders & lower back)

Considerations: surface of pool floor, depth and level of water.

Alternatives: overhead hoist and sling with floating tabs, or change seat attachment to hoist to a spreader bar attachment to use with slings (discuss with manufacturer). Child secured in wheeled shower chair and wheeled down sloping access into pool.

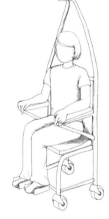

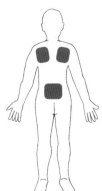 Areas of potential handler discomfort

40 Transfer into pool - stretcher/flat bed hoist

Child in swimsuit hoisted to pool stretcher and then into pool. Handler in pool assists child to float off when in water.

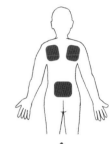

Child ability	**1 - 3**

Child size: C - F
Child comfort: 8

 Hoist and sling to position child on flat bed pool stretcher.

Handler effort: **11 - 13**
Risk to handler: **low**
(shoulders & lower back)

Considerations: child behaviour and ability to keep still during transfer. Sufficient time must be allowed for task.

Alternatives: supportive sling on special spreader bar on pool hoist, child secured in wheeled shower chair and wheeled down sloping access to pool.

● A handler must be in water to receive child.

Areas of potential handler discomfort

Horse riding

41 Helping larger more able person onto horse

Larger, more able, young person can be assisted to mount from standing. They stand on mounting block or raised ramp and handler assists by placing one of rider's feet into the stirrup and their other leg over horse. Second handler guides from other side.

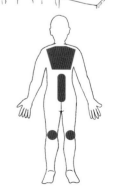

Child ability	**5 - 7**

Child size: D - F
Child comfort: 7

 Mounting block, raised ramp.

Handler effort: **13**
Risk to handler: **medium/high**
(lumbar spine, knees & shoulders)

● Third handler steadies the horse

Considerations: young person's weight, height, standing ability and predictability of their co-operation. Predictability of horse.

Alternatives: use hoist, assist young person into pony and trap, computer simulation on mechanical 'horse'. Assisting child to lie over saddle and be assisted into sitting, or lying on tummy facing horse's tail. Note: there are various different options for horse riding and not all are covered in this book. Physio/occupational therapist, manual handling practitioner or local Riding for the Disabled group may be able to offer further advice.

Areas of potential handler discomfort

42 Hoisting child onto horse

Child is hoisted from seated position in chair beside horse, using either standard sling, access sling or walking harness. They are then positioned to raise a leg over saddle while second person helps/adjusts from other side.

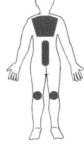

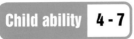 **Child ability** | **4 - 7**

Child size: **B - F**
Child comfort: **5**

 Overhead tracking suitable sling.

Handler effort: **13**
Risk to handler: **medium**
(shoulders, lumbar spine & knees)

Considerations: child's weight, size, muscle tone, involuntary movements, and stability. Predictability of horse.

Alternatives: usually considered the safer option for helping child onto horse. A child with some weight-bearing ability can be helped onto mounting block and 'flopped' face-down over saddle, then leg nearest horse's tail is lifted over the saddle. Special saddles may be used for some children, or some may lie on horse's back facing tail.

● Third handler steadies the horse

 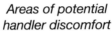

Areas of potential handler discomfort

Tricycles

43 Helping weightbearing child onto trike

Helping child from standing on floor onto saddle of bike by standing transfer, with child lifting (may require assistance) nearside leg across frame.

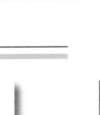

Child ability | **3 - 6**

Child size: **C - E**
Child comfort: **6**

 Small step often required, suitably modified tricycle with saddle supports and pedal footstraps, chock or brakes to stabilise trike.

Handler effort: **15**
Risk to handler: **medium**
(lumar spine & knees)

Considerations: technique should not be used for NON weight-bearing children. Important that handlers know which trike parts can be moved and that it is right size for child. Handler assisting may often have difficulty helping child and attaching straps, so two people required.

Alternatives: different trike design, hoisting with full body sling or standing harness.

● Third handler may be needed to steady trike.

Areas of potential handler discomfort

---

44 Hoisting child onto trike

Using a standard sling and suitable hoist/overhead tracking to lift child onto trike.

Child ability **3 - 4**

Child size: **B - F**
Child comfort: **8**

 Hoist which fits around trike and raises high enough/overhead tracking. Trike with side supports to saddle which swing away.

Handler effort: **10**
Risk to handler: **low**
(shoulders, lower back & wrists)

Considerations: planning required as not all hoist/sling combinations will work. There must be enough height clearance between hoist and trike, so mobile hoist may not work for larger children. Risk of straps being caught in wheels/pedals.

Alternatives: standing transfer with walking harness. Different style of trike.

⚠ *Areas of potential handler discomfort*

● Third handler may be needed to hold trike.

Trampolines

45 Transfer child onto high trampoline

Hoisting child/young person onto raised trampoline from wheelchair.

Child ability **1 - 3**

Child size: **C - F**
Child comfort: **8**

 Large mobile hoist with high lift capability, suitable sling, slide sheet(s) to move child to centre of trampoline.

  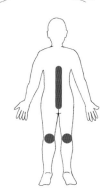

Handler effort: **13**
Risk to handler: **medium**
(lumbar spine & knees)

Considerations: child's weight, height, unpredictability of movement, muscle tone, anxiety; ceiling height as tracking not usually permissible over trampolines.

Alternatives: use trampoline at floor level – with pit beneath. Tracking and use of gantry may cause problems over any trampoline due to possibility of children hitting their heads on it.

⚠ *Areas of potential handler discomfort*

46 Transferring child to floor level trampoline

Hoisting child from chair to floor adjacent to trampoline surface, sliding them over edge on slide sheets.

 Child ability | **1 - 3**

Child size: **A - D**
Child comfort: **6**

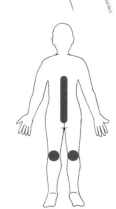

 Mobile hoist, sling, two to three flat slide sheets.

Handler effort: **13**
Risk to handler: **medium**
(lumbar spine & knees)

Considerations: stability of floor, skill of handlers on trampoline, unpredictable movements of child. Overhead tracking or portable gantry hoist may not be safe due to ceiling height. Larger children will be difficult to pull back, due to weight, on trampoline.

Alternatives: use pool type hoist, as long as the hoist mast is sufficiently clear of bouncing children.

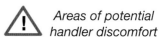

Areas of potential handler discomfort

47 Transfer to floor level trampoline - special hoist

Hoisting child from chair onto trampoline.

 Child ability | **1 - 3**

Child size: **C - F**
Child comfort: **6**

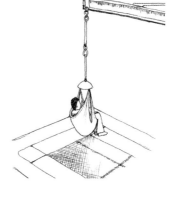

Special floor-mounted hoist with extended boom, sling.

Handler effort: **11**
Risk to handler: **medium**
(lumbar spine & knees)

Considerations: stability of floor, skill of handlers on trampoline, unpredictability of child's movements.

Alternatives: some venues may not have sufficient height above trampoline surface to allow for use of gantry or tracking hoist. Consider another venue.

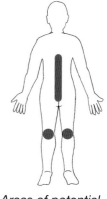

Areas of potential handler discomfort

Transport

Children with mobility impairments often require assisted transport to school, or for family outings. Some can be assisted into car seat or booster, others may require seats which swing out to avoid handlers stretching into car. Some car seats have swivel bases to reduce twisting involved.

Many children travel in their wheelchairs in wheelchair accessible vehicles. It is essential their wheelchair is restrained, as well using the seat belt on the child as required by law. A posture belt is not sufficient protection.

Some vehicles have passenger lifts, others have ramps and may have winches to assist in pulling chairs up slopes into vehicles.

48 Transfer onto minibus - child who can stand

Helping child who can perform standing transfer onto minibus. Child uses passenger lift to ascend into vehicle, is then assisted to stand from wheelchair and to turn and sit on bus seat.

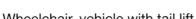 **Child ability** **5 - 7**

Child size: **C - F**
Child comfort: **8**

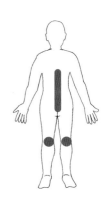

 Wheelchair, vehicle with tail lift.

  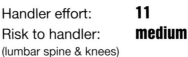

Handler effort: **11**
Risk to handler: **medium**
(lumbar spine & knees)

Considerations: predictability and co-operation of child will significantly affect this transfer, as handler will rely on them needing minimal assistance. Width of aisle and whether child needs to move to a window seat can make this transfer more difficult, as will be case if child needs to use booster seat.

Alternatives: child travels in wheelchair in bus with suitable wheelchair restraints and seat belt.

⚠ *Areas of potential handler discomfort*

49 Assisting small child into car seat

Child is lifted from push chair/seat and into car seat by handler stepping into car with one foot. The relevant straps are then secured.

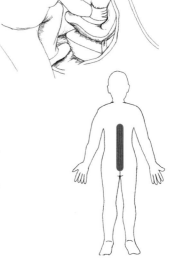

| Child ability | 1 - 3 |

Child size: A - B
Child comfort: 9

 Car and booster seat.

Handler effort: **12**
Risk to handler: **medium**
(lumbar spine)

Considerations: Although each individual lift may be medium risk, consider cumulative effects, especially for the more dependent child. Weight of child, height of car roof – as this may restrict posture – type of child seat, width of car door opening (or of minibus aisle), which seat is used (on double seats). unpredictablity/involuntary movements of small child.

Alternatives: for a child needing support while placed in seat and strapped, try specialised car seat which swivels. To avoid stoop and twist, use 'crash tested' wheel chair for transport in a suitable vehicle.

⚠ *Areas of potential handler discomfort*

50 Non-weightbearing wheelchair user onto bus

Using passenger lift to ascend to vehicle with wheelchair brakes applied, or using ramps into vehicle – perhaps with winch. Handler usually accompanies child on lift if sufficient room. If not, second handler receives child at top.

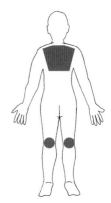

| Child ability | 1 - 4 |

Child size: B - F
Child comfort: 10

 Ramps or vehicle passenger lift.

Handler effort: **13**
Risk to handler: **medium**
(shoulders & knees)

Considerations: type of ramp or lift will affect effort required for this task and whether handler can travel on lift with child (due to lift size); headroom inside vehicle, complexity of clamping and seat belt system, space available.

Alternatives: wheelchair accessible black cab.

⚠ *Areas of potential handler discomfort*

A practical problem solving tool

The following table has been compiled as a problem solving tool and includes some of the data taken from the individual tasks. It is intended to provide a quick guide to help handlers (having estimated a child's size and ability) to decide on the available range of tasks as listed in the book and the level of risk to themselves. It will direct readers to a particular page for further information. Some tasks have a low, medium and high risk option, but high risk options are not listed for all tasks.

The handler/assessor can also use the table for children who are new to them, or their establishments, to help develop a plan or strategy.

> Note: risk level shown in chart is lowest to the handler as assessed by the authors. The actual risk may be higher depending on individual circumstances.

Example: Sophie is due to start a new school. The SENCO/INCO there has been told that Sophie is child size D (D = Older children 7 - 12

years estimated weight range 26-35 kg) and that she can stand but gradually sags at the knees.

They have assessed Sophie's ability score as 3 (moderate assistance, performs 50-74% of task) but because of her sagging – and without any equipment at the old school – she has been lifted onto a change table by two people to assist with personal care.

Looking at the chart for child size D, there are 4 options listed for Sophie. Two low risk tasks (Tasks 3, 6) and 2 medium risk tasks (7 and 10).

The SENCO/INCO can then turn to the relevant pages in this publication, and use the information as a discussion point to choose the best option for Sophie.

It may highlight that personal care needs to be reviewed, require further discussion, or have equipment and staff implications.

The limited information in the table should never be used in isolation to perform a task, but with reference to the full text and with careful discussion with all parties concerned – including the child wherever possible.

Child size A – handler risk table

Risk key ■ low   ▧ medium   ▨ high   ■ very high   (Task number background colour indicates risk level)

Child ability	Risk/task no	Task description	Page
Floorwork			
4-5	22	Transfer partly weight bearing child to buggy from low seat/floor	56
1	27	Manual lift small child from low surface	58
1	28	Lift from floor using lifting sling	59
1-2	25	Transfer to buggy/corner or low seat to or from floor	57
3-5	23	Helping to stand – from lap	56
Personal care			
3-5	6	Hoisting child from chair to toilet using access sling	46
1-7	8	Lifting child to changing table	47
Therapy transfer			
1-4	34	Manual transfer to/from ball	63
Pools			
3-5	38	Transfer small child to swimming/therapy pool	65
Trampoline			
1-3	46	Transfer to floor-level trampoline	69
Transport			
1-3	49	Helping small child into car seat	71

Risk key ▬ low ▬ medium ▬ high ▬ very high (Task number background colour indicates risk level)

Child size B – handler risk table

Child ability	Risk/task no		Task description	Page
Floorwork	1-5	26	Hoisting child to/from floor	58
	4-5	22	Transfer partial weightbearing child to buggy or low seat	56
	1	27	Manual lift small child from low surface	58
	1	28	Lift from floor using lifting sling	59
	1-2	25	Transfer to/from buggy corner/low seat to from floor	57
	3-5	23	Helping to standing (from lap)	56
Horse riding	4-7	42	Hoisting child onto horse	67
Personal care	3-5	6	Hoisting from chair to toilet using access sling	46
	5-6	5	Toilet transfer with portable step	45
	1-4	10	Hoist to change table for personal care	48
	2-5	9	Two people lifting child to changing table	48
	5-7	1	Help standing child to change pad	43
	1-7	8	Lift child to changing table	47
Showering/ bathing	1-2	12	Showering on wheeled seat/commode	49
	1-4	13	Showering using shower trolley	50
	1-4	14	Help child to roll	50
Standing & walking	3-4	20	Help to walk with walking harness	54
	4-6	18	Help to walk with walking frame	53
	5-6	17	Help to walk with wheelie stool	52
	5-7	15	Help from sit to stand	51
Standing frame/therapy transfers	1-5	32	Hoisting to supine standing frame/tilt table	62
	3-5	35	Hoisting to a wedge	63
	1-2	37	Manual turn onto wedge/side lier on floor	64
	1-4	34	Manual transfer to/from ball	63
	2-5	33	Hoist to/from ball	62
	3-4	36	Supported sitting	64
	3-7	30	Helping seated child into upright stander	60
Pools	3-5	38	Helping small child into swimming/therapy pool	65
Trampoline	1-3	46	Transfer to floor-level trampoline	69
Transport	1-4	50	Helping non-weightbearing wheelchair-user onto bus	71
	1-3	49	Helping small child into car seat	71
Tricycle	3-4	44	Hoisting onto trike	68

Child size C – handler risk table

Child ability	Risk/task no	Task description	Page
Floorwork			
1-5	26	Hoisting child to/from floor	58
4-6	24	Using inflatable raiser cushion to help child on/off floor	57
5-7	21	Off floor (independent)	55
Horse riding			
4-7	42	Hoisting child on/off horse	67
Personal care			
3-5	6	Hoisting from chair to toilet using access sling	46
5-6	5	Toilet transfer with portable raised step	45
5-7	2	Helping standing child (usually a boy) to use uriine bottle	44
1-4	10	Hoisting to change table for personal care	48
2-5	9	Two people lifting to change table	48
5-7	1	Helping standing child change pad	43
Showering/ bathing			
1-2	12	Showering on wheeled seat/commode	49
1-4	13	Showering using shower trolley	50
1-4	14	Help child to roll	50
5-7	11	Showering child on pull-down seat	49
Standing & walking			
3-4	20	Help to walk with walking harness	54
4-6	18	Help to walk with walking frame	53
5-6	17	Help to walk with wheelie stool	52
5-7	19	Stand and turn aid	53
5-7	15	Help from sit to stand	51
5-7	16	Help from sit to stand (additional help from side if required)	52
Standing frame/therapy transfers			
1-5	32	Hoisting to supine standing frame/tilt table	62
2-7	31	Hoisting into prone standing frame	61
3-5	35	Hoisting onto a wedge	63
1-2	37	Manually turning child onto wedge/side lier on floor	64
1-4	34	Manual transfer to/from ball	63
2-5	33	Hoist to/from ball	62
3-4	36	Supported sitting	64
3-7	30	Helping seated child into upright stander	60
5-7	29	Partial weightbearer into prone/upright stander from change bed	60
Pools			
2	40	Hoist into pool using stretcher/flatbed hoist	66
Trampoline			
1-3	45	Helping child onto high trampoline	68
1-3	46	Transfer to floor-level trampoline	69
1-3	47	Transfer larger child to floor-level trampoline with special hoist	69
Transport			
1-4	50	Taking non-weightbearing wheelchair-user onto bus	71
5-7	48	Helping child (able to perform standing transfer) onto minibus	70
Tricycle			
3-4	44	Hoisting onto trike	68
3-6	43	Helping weightbearing child onto trike	67

Child size D **Risk key** low medium high very high (Task number background colour indicates risk level)

	Child ability	Risk/task no	Task description	Page
Floorwork	1-5	26	Hoisting child to/from floor	58
	4-6	24	Using inflatable raiser cushion to help child on/off floor	57
	5-7	21	Off floor (independent)	55
Horse riding	4-7	42	Hoisting child on/off horse	67
	5-7	41	Helping larger more able person on/off horse	66
Personal care	3-5	3	Helping child in chair use urine bottle	44
	3-5	6	Hoisting from chair to toilet using access sling	46
	5-6	5	Toilet transfer with portable raised step	45
	5-7	4	Using transfer board to move from one seated position to another	45
	1-4	10	Hoisting child to change table for personal care	48
	2-4	7	Helping child in sling use urine bottle	47
	5-7	1	Helping standing child change pad	43
Showering/ bathing	1-2	12	Showering on wheeled seat/commode	49
	1-4	13	Showering using shower trolley	50
	1-4	14	Helping child to roll	50
	5-7	11	Showering child on pull-down seat	49
Standing & walking	3-4	20	Help to walk with walking harness	54
	4-6	18	Helping child walk with walking frame	53
	5-7	19	Stand and turn aid	53
	5-7	15	Help from sit to stand	51
	5-7	16	Help from sit to stand (additional help from side if required)	52
Standing frame/therapy transfers	1-5	32	Hoisting onto supine standing frame/tilt table	62
	2-7	31	Hoisting into prone standing frame	61
	3-5	35	Hoisting on/off a wedge	63
	1-2	37	Manually turning child onto wedge/side lier on floor	64
	2-5	33	Hoist to/from ball	62
	3-7	30	Transfer seated child into upright stander	60
	5-7	29	Partial weightbearer into prone/upright stander from change bed	60
Pools	2	40	Hoist into pool using stretcher/flatbed hoist	66
	4-7	39	Hoist into pool using pool chair	65
Trampoline	1-3	45	Helping child onto high trampoline	68
	1-3	46	Transfer to floor-level trampoline	69
	1-3	47	Transfer larger child to floor-level trampoline with special hoist	69
Transport	1-4	50	Taking non-weightbearing wheelchair-user onto bus	71
	5-7	48	Helping child (able to perform standing transfer) onto minibus	70
Tricycle	3-4	44	Hoisting onto trike	68
	3-6	43	Helping weightbearing child onto trike	67

Risk key ▇ low ▨ medium ▨ high █ very high (Task number background colour indicates risk level)

Child size E – handler risk table

Child ability		Risk/task no	Task description	Page
Floorwork	1-5	26	Hoisting child to/from floor	58
	4-6	24	Using inflatable raiser cushion to help child to/from floor	57
	5-7	21	Off floor (independent)	55
Horse riding	4-7	42	Hoisting child onto horse	67
	5-7	41	Helping larger, more able person, who can be assisted, onto horse	66
Personal care	3-5	3	Helping child in chair use urine bottle	44
	3-5	6	Hoisting from chair to toilet using access sling	46
	5-7	4	Using transfer board to move from one seated position to another	45
	1-4	10	Hoist to change table for personal care	48
	2-4	7	Helping child in sling use urine bottle	47
	5-7	1	Help standing child to change pad	43
Showering/ bathing	1-2	12	Showering on wheeled seat/commode	49
	1-4	13	Showering using shower trolley	50
	1-4	14	Help child to roll	50
	5-7	11	Showering child on pull-down seat	49
Standing & walking	3-4	20	Help to walk with walking harness	54
	4-6	18	Help to walk with walking frame	53
	5-7	19	Stand and turn aid	53
	5-7	15	Help from sit to stand	51
	5-7	16	Sit to stand from front (with additional help from side if required	52
Standing frame/therapy transfers	1-5	32	Hoisting to supine standing frame/tilt table	62
	2-7	31	Hoisting child into prone standing frame	61
	2-5	33	Hoist to/from ball	62
	3-7	30	Transferring seated child into upright stander	60
	5-7	29	Partial weightbearer into prone/upright stander from change bed	60
Pools	2	40	Hoist transfer to pool using stretcher/flat-bed hoist	66
	4-7	39	Hoist transfer to pool using pool chair	65
Trampoline	1-3	45	Transfer child onto high trampoline	68
	1-3	47	Transfer larger child to floor-level trampoline with special hoist	69
Transport	1-4	50	Helping non-weightbearing wheelchair-user onto bus	71
	5-7	48	Helping wheelchair user (able to do standing transfer) onto minibus	70
Tricycle	3-4	44	Hoisting onto trike	68
	3-6	43	Helping weightbearing child onto trike	67

Risk key   ▨ low   ▨ medium   ▨ high   ▨ very high   (Task number background colour indicates risk level)

Child size F – handler risk table

Child ability	Child ability (range)	Risk/task no	Task description	Page
Floorwork	1-5	26	Hoisting child to/from floor	58
	4-6	24	Using inflatable raiser cushion to help child to/from floor	57
	5-7	21	Off floor (independent)	55
Horse riding	4-7	42	Hoisting child onto horse	67
	5-7	41	Helping larger, more able person, who can be assisted, onto horse	66
Personal care	3-5	3	Helping child in chair use urine bottle	44
	3-5	6	Hoisting from chair to toilet using access sling	46
	5-7	4	Using transfer board to move from one seated position to another	45
	1-4	10	Hoist to change table for personal care	48
	2-4	7	Helping child in sling use urine bottle	47
Showering/ bathing	1-2	12	Showering on wheeled seat/commode	49
	1-4	13	Showering using shower trolley	50
	1-4	14	Help child to roll	50
	5-7	11	Showering child on pull-down seat	49
Standing & walking	3-4	20	Help to walk with walking harness	54
	4-6	18	Help to walk with walking frame	53
	5-7	19	Stand and turn aid	53
	5-7	15	Help from sit to stand	51
	5-7	16	Sit to stand from front (with additional help from side if required)	52
Standing frame/therapy transfers	1-5	32	Hoisting to supine standing frame/tilt table	62
	2-7	31	Hoisting child into prone standing frame	61
	2-5	33	Hoist to/from ball	62
	3-7	30	Transferring seated child into upright stander	60
Pools	2	40	Hoist transfer to pool using stretcher/flat-bed hoist	66
	4-7	39	Hoist transfer to pool using pool chair	65
Trampoline	1-3	45	Transfer child onto high trampoline	68
	1-3	47	Transfer larger child to floor-level trampoline with special hoist	69
Transport	1-4	50	Helping non-weightbearing wheelchair-user onto bus	71
	3-4	48	Helping child (able to perform standing transfer) onto minibus	70
Tricycle	3-4	44	Hoisting onto trike	68

References

A&B, X&Y v East Sussex County Council (2003) EWHC 167 (Admin) High Court: paragraphs 128/129 (Neutral Citation Number: [2003] EWHC 167 (Admin)).

Association of Paediatric Chartered Physiotherapists (1998), Paediatric Manual Handling Guidelines for Paediatric Physiotherapists: ACPC.

Benner, P (1984) From Novice to Expert: Excellence and power in clinical nursing practice. Menlo Park: Addison-Wesley.

Borg, G (1998) Perceived Exertion and Pain Scales, United Graphics, USA.

Critchon, N (2001) Visual Analogue Scales (VAS) Journal of Clinical Nursing, 10, pp 697-706, Blackwell Science Ltd.

Department for Education and Skills (2004) Every Child Matters – change for children, DfES: Nottingham.

Devon County Council (2006) Guidance for staff who provide intimate care for children and young people – including a model policy published by DCC, April 2006.

Dreyfus, L & Dreyfus, SE (1986) Mind Over Machine: The Power of Human Intuition and Expertise in the Era of the Computer, Blackwell: Oxford.

Equality Act, 2010, http://www.legislation.gov.uk/ukpga/2010/15/pdfs/ukpga_20100015_en.pdf

Granger, CV., Hamilton, BB., Linacre, JM., Heinemann, AW. and Wright, BD (1993) Performance Profiles of Functional Independence Measure, Am J Phys Med Rehabilitation, 72: 84-9.

Health and Safety at Work etc Act. (1974) http://www.hse.govuk/legislation/hswa

Health and Safety Executive (1998) Safe use of lifting equipment. Lifting Operations and Lifting Equipment Regulations, L113. Suffolk: HSE Books.

Health and Safety Executive (1998a) Safe use of work equipment. Provision and Use of Work Equipment Regulations. L22 (2nd edition) Suffolk: HSE Books.

Health and Safety Executive (2001) Handling Home Care, HMSO: Norwich.

Health and Safety Executive (2004) Manual Handling Operations Regulations 1992 (as amended) Guidance on Regulations L23 (3rd edition) Suffolk: HSE Books.

Health and Safety Executive (2006) Five Steps to Risk Assessment, Suffolk: HSE Books.

Hull, D and Johnston D (1999) Essential Paediatrics (4th edition) Elsevier.

Likert, R (1932) A Technique for the Measurement of Attitudes, Archives of Psychology 140: 1-55.

National Back Exchange (2003) Position Statement in physically assisting people – making balanced decisions, Column, August 15.3 p5.

National Patient Safety Association (2008) A Risk Matrix for Managers, NPSA, London.

Ruszala, S., Hall, J. and Alexander, P (2010) Standards in Manual Handling (3rd edition) National Back Exchange: Towcester.

Scotland's Commissioner for Children and Young People (2008) Handle with Care, SCCYP: Edinburgh.

Smith, J (2011) The Guide to the Handling of People, a systems approach (6th edition) BackCare, Teddington.

Townsend, P (2010) Paediatric Manual Handling – meeting complex needs, Column, Winter 22.1 pp16-18.

USDAW (2009) Body mapping – Telling Where it Hurts, http://www.usdaw.org.uk/healthandsafety